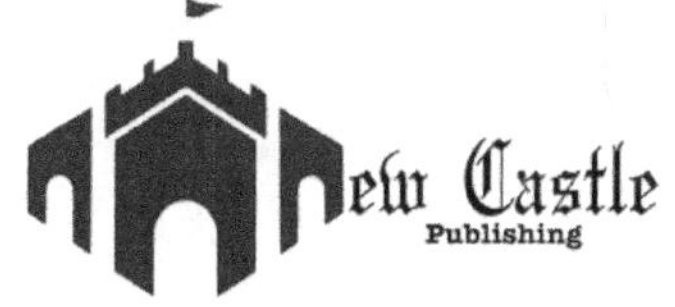

New Castle
Publishing

Fitness Decoded

Unlocking the Secrets to a Healthiness, & Happiness at any Age!

By

Kevin DiBacco

Copyright 2024 by Kevin DiBacco

All rights reserved. No part of this book may be reproduced in any form
or by any means without the prior written consent of the Publisher,
excepting brief quotes used in reviews.
This book is registered at the U.S. Patent and Trademark Offices.

Cover design © 2024 Yellowdogdigitalstudios. All rights reserved.

DISCLAIMER

No part of this publication may be reproduced in any form or by any
means, including printing, scanning, photocopying, or otherwise,

without the prior written permission of the copyright holder. The author has tried to present information that is as correct and concrete as possible. The author is not a medical doctor and does not write in any medical capacity. All medical decisions should be made under the guidance and care of your primary physician. The author will not be held liable for any injury or loss that is incurred to the reader through the application of the information here contained in this book. The author emphasizes that the medical field is fast evolving with newer studies being done continuously, therefore the information in this book is only a researched collaboration of accurate information at the time of writing. With the ever-changing nature of the subjects included, the author hopes that the reader will be able to appreciate the content that has been covered in this book. While all attempts have been made to verify each piece of information provided in this publication, the author assumes no responsibility for any error, omission, or contrary interpretation of the subject present in this book. Please note that any help or advice given hereof is not a substitution for licensed medical advice. The reader accepts responsibility in the use of any information and takes advice given in this book at their own risk. If the reader is under medication supervision or has had complications with health-related risks, consult your primary care physician as soon as possible before taking any advice given in this book.

"The information and advice contained in this book are based upon the research and the personal and professional experiences of the author. They are not intended as a substitute for consulting a healthcare professional. The publisher and author are not

Contents

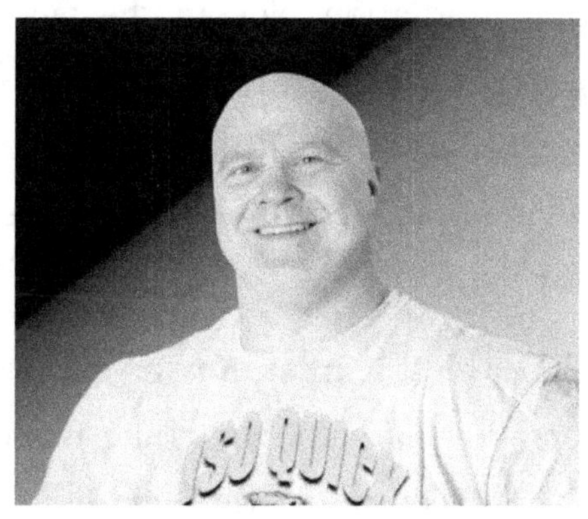

About the Author

Kevin DiBacco is a true renaissance man whose life journey embodies the spirit of resilience, determination, and continuous growth. His multifaceted career spans competitive powerlifting, filmmaking, and authorship, each chapter of his life marked by remarkable achievements and unwavering perseverance in the face of adversity.

For 20 years, Kevin dominated the world of competitive powerlifting, honing not just his physical strength but also the mental fortitude that would serve him throughout his life. This foundation in athletics laid the groundwork for his philosophy of pushing beyond perceived limits and never backing down from a challenge.

Kevin's journey, however, has been far from smooth. His medical history reads like an orthopedic textbook: 6 knee operations, 2 major back surgeries, 2 hip replacements, brain surgery, and brain radiation. Yet, in the face of these daunting health challenges, Kevin's spirit remained unbroken. At the age of 62, he embarked on a monumental fitness journey, shedding 60 pounds and proving that age is merely a number when it comes to personal transformation.

Following his athletic career, Kevin ventured into the world of filmmaking. For 37 remarkable years, he worked as a filmmaker and video producer, securing 5 worldwide film distribution deals. His experience in visualizing and executing complex film projects would later influence his approach to writing and personal development.

Today, Kevin DiBacco is a bestselling author, using his gift for storytelling to inspire and motivate readers around the world. He is the author of several acclaimed books, including:

- "HYSOMETRICS"

- "Indie Filmmaking in the REAL WORLD"

- "Hold the Power"

- "The Handshake around the World"

- "The Lost Art of Logical Thinking"

- "Recharge: The Powernap"

- "Chemicals in our food: What's really on your plate?"

His biography, "The Gabardine Gang," further cements his status as a versatile and engaging author.

Drawing from his vast experience and the lessons learned through his personal challenges, Kevin developed "ISO QUICK STRENGTH," a program designed to help people rebound after setbacks. He recognized that overcoming difficulties requires both physical and mental strength, a principle that permeates all of his work.

Kevin is also a firm believer in the power of visualization, a technique he has used throughout his diverse career. From powerlifting competitions to film productions to writing books, his motto "If you can see it, you can do it" has been a guiding principle.

Known as the "Life Warrior," Kevin embodies the philosophy that one must be "willing to do whatever it takes to overcome life's challenges." His personal mantra, "Those who quit will always fail," encapsulates the indomitable spirit that has carried him through numerous obstacles and setbacks.

Through his blog, books, and personal example, Kevin continues to spread his message of resilience and determination. His journey stands as a testament to the human capacity for overcoming adversity and the power of embracing life's challenges with an open heart and warrior spirit.

Kevin DiBacco's life story is one of courage, adaptability, and relentless pursuit of growth. Whether on the powerlifting platform, behind the camera, or at the writing desk, he continues to inspire others to push beyond their limits and embrace the warrior within.

Unlocking the Secrets to a Healthiness, & Happiness at any Age!

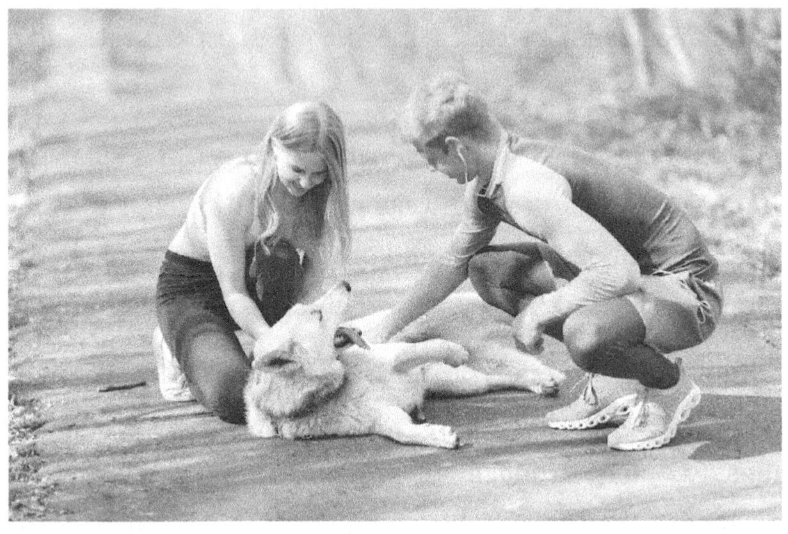

The journey to fitness is not a straight path. It's a winding road filled with challenges, setbacks, and moments of triumph. This book acknowledges this reality, offering not just exercises and diet plans, but a comprehensive toolkit for navigating the complexities of a fitness journey. It recognizes that true, lasting change comes not just from knowing what to do, but from understanding why we do it and how to sustain it.

What I find particularly commendable about this work is its accessibility. Whether you're taking your first tentative steps towards a healthier lifestyle or you're a seasoned athlete looking to break through plateaus, you'll find value in these pages. The author's approach is both compassionate and practical, acknowledging the struggles we all face while providing actionable steps to overcome them.

This book delves deep into the psychological aspects of fitness, offering insights that go beyond the physical. It challenges readers to rethink their relationship with their bodies, their health, and ultimately, themselves. By fostering a positive fitness mindset, readers will find themselves not just meeting their health goals but exceeding them in ways they never thought possible.

In a world that often prioritizes quick fixes and instant gratification, "Fitness Decoded" stands as a testament to the power of sustainable change. It reminds us that lasting transformation comes from within, and that with the right mindset and tools, we all have the power to rewrite our health narratives.

As you embark on this journey through the pages of "Fitness Decoded," I encourage you to approach it with an open heart and mind. Allow yourself to be challenged, to question long-held beliefs, and to envision a version of yourself that is stronger, healthier, and more fulfilled than ever before.

Remember, true fitness is not a destination, but a lifelong journey of growth and self-discovery. This book is not just a guide, but a companion on that journey. It offers the knowledge, strategies, and motivation to help you unlock your full potential and achieve a level of health and happiness you may have thought unattainable.

So, take a deep breath, turn the page, and prepare to embark on a transformative journey. Your path to decoding fitness and unlocking a healthier, happier you start here. Embrace the challenge, celebrate the victories, and get ready to redefine what fitness means to you.

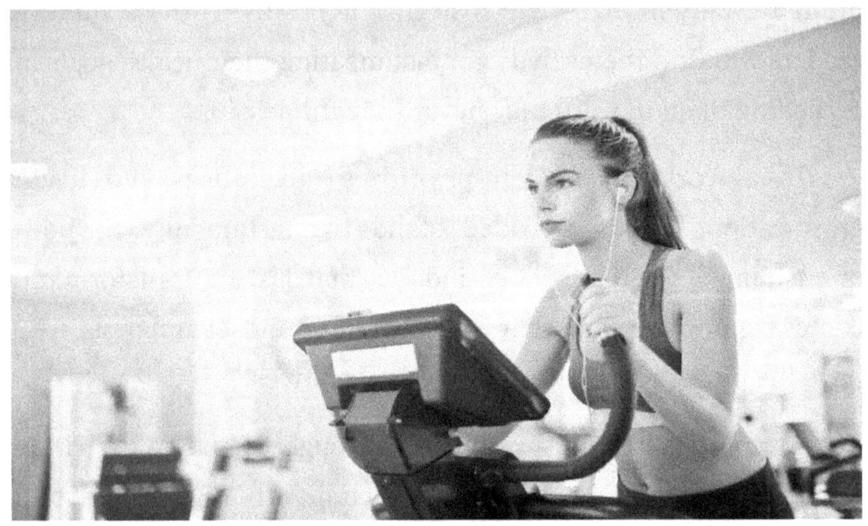

Introduction

The Importance of Fitness in Modern Life

In the tapestry of modern existence, fitness stands out as a crucial thread, weaving its way through every aspect of our lives. Far from being a mere luxury or a pursuit of the aesthetically inclined, fitness has emerged as a fundamental pillar of well-being in our fast-paced, often stressful world. But what exactly do we mean by fitness, and why has it become so vital in our contemporary society?

Fitness, in its broadest sense, encompasses not just physical strength and endurance, but also mental acuity, emotional balance, and overall vitality. It's about cultivating a state of being that allows us to meet the demands of daily life with energy and enthusiasm, while also building resilience against the myriad challenges we face.

In our sedentary, technology-driven era, the importance of physical fitness cannot be overstated. Our bodies, evolved for movement and physical exertion, often find themselves at odds with our modern lifestyles. Hours spent hunched over desks, eyes fixed on screens, have led to a host of health issues – from obesity and cardiovascular diseases to chronic back pain and mental health disorders. Regular physical activity serves as a powerful antidote to these modern maladies, helping to maintain healthy body weight, improve cardiovascular health, strengthen muscles and bones, and boost overall immune function.

But the benefits of fitness extend far beyond the physical realm. In a world where mental health challenges are on the rise, the psychological benefits of fitness have come into sharp focus. Exercise has been shown to be a potent mood elevator, releasing endorphins that combat stress, anxiety, and depression. Regular physical activity improves sleep quality, enhances cognitive function, and boosts self-esteem – all crucial components of mental well-being.

Moreover, fitness plays a vital role in our social connections. In an age where digital interactions often replace face-to-face contact, fitness activities – whether it's a group exercise class, a team sport, or a hiking club – provide opportunities for real-world social engagement. These connections not only enhance our enjoyment of physical activities but also contribute to our overall sense of community and belonging.

From a broader perspective, the importance of fitness extends to societal and economic realms. A fit population is generally a more productive one, with lower healthcare costs and higher quality of life. As we grapple with global challenges like rising healthcare expenses and an aging population, promoting fitness becomes not just a personal imperative but a societal one.

Yet, despite its undeniable importance, many of us struggle to make fitness a priority in our lives. We're bombarded with conflicting information, fad diets, and extreme workout regimens that often do more harm than good. We set unrealistic goals, get discouraged by slow progress, or simply feel overwhelmed by the prospect of change. This is where the concept of "decoding" fitness becomes crucial – and it's what this book is all about.

Overview of the Book's Structure and Goals

"**Fitness Decoded**: Unlocking the Secrets to a Healthier, Happier You" is designed to be your compass in the often-confusing world of health and fitness. Our goal is not to provide yet another set of exercises or diet plans (though we'll certainly cover these). Instead, we aim to help you understand the underlying principles of fitness, empowering you to make informed decisions and develop sustainable habits that lead to lasting health and happiness.

This book is structured to take you on a transformative journey, divided into several key chapters:

1. **The Foundations of Fitness**: We'll explore the basic components of fitness, including cardiovascular health, strength training, flexibility, and nutrition. This chapter will provide a solid understanding of what constitutes a well-rounded fitness program.

2. **The Science of Exercise**: Delve into the physiological and biochemical processes that occur in our bodies during and after exercise. Understanding the 'why' behind fitness can be a powerful motivator.

3. **Nutrition Demystified**: Navigate the often-confusing world of nutrition. Learn about macronutrients, micronutrients, and how to create a balanced diet that supports your fitness goals.

4. **The Psychology of Fitness**: Explore the mental aspects of fitness, including motivation, goal setting, and overcoming psychological barriers. Discover how to develop a mindset that supports long-term success.

5. **Customizing Your Fitness Journey**: Learn how to create a fitness plan that's tailored to your individual needs, preferences, and lifestyle. Understand how to adapt your approach as your fitness level improves or as life circumstances change.

6. **Recovery and Injury Prevention**: Discover the crucial role of rest and recovery in any fitness program. Learn techniques for preventing injuries and how to listen to your body's signals.

7. **Fitness Technology and Tools**: Navigate the world of fitness apps, wearables, and other technological aids. Learn how to use these tools effectively without becoming overly dependent on them.

8. **Maintaining Long-Term Success**: Develop strategies for making fitness a lifelong habit. Learn how to overcome plateaus, stay motivated, and continually challenge yourself.

9. **Fitness Myths Debunked**: Separate fact from fiction in the world of fitness. We'll address common misconceptions and provide evidence-based information to guide your choices.

10.

11.   **Integrating Fitness into Your Lifestyle**: Discover how to make fitness an integral part of your daily life, rather than a separate obligation. Learn to find joy in movement and to see opportunities for activity in everyday situations.

Throughout these chapters, you'll find not just theoretical concepts, but practical exercises, real-life examples, and actionable strategies. Our goal is to empower you with the knowledge and tools to not just start your fitness journey, but to sustain it for life.

Remember, this book is not about achieving perfection or adhering to rigid standards. It's about progress, self-compassion, and the joy of discovering what your body and mind are capable of. It's about finding a balance that works for you, and about viewing fitness not as a destination, but as a lifelong adventure.

As we embark on this journey together, I invite you to approach each chapter with an open mind and a willingness to challenge your preconceptions about fitness and health. By the time you turn the last page, my hope is that you'll not only have a clear understanding of what it takes to be fit and healthy, but also a newfound excitement for the path ahead.

Let's begin this transformative journey towards decoding fitness and unlocking a healthier, happier you. Welcome to "Fitness Decoded: Unlocking the Secrets to a Healthier, Happier You."

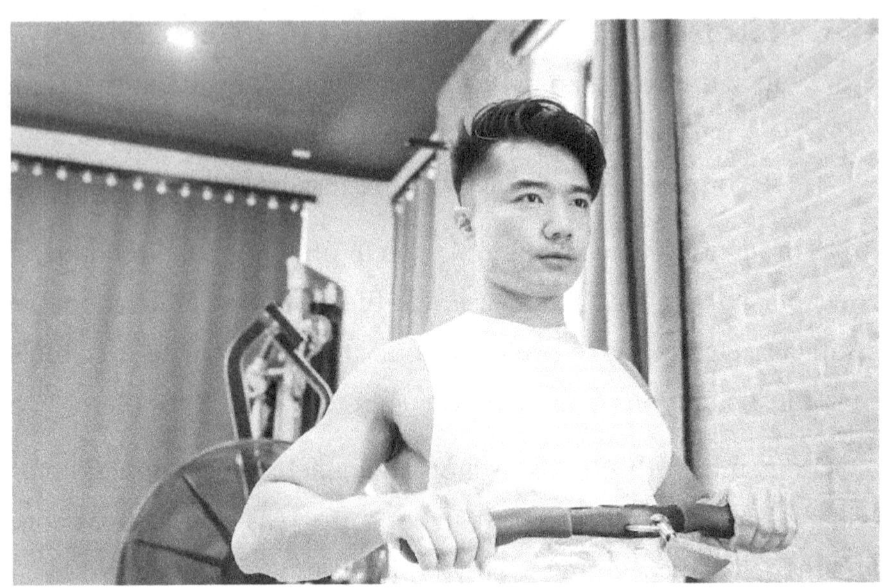

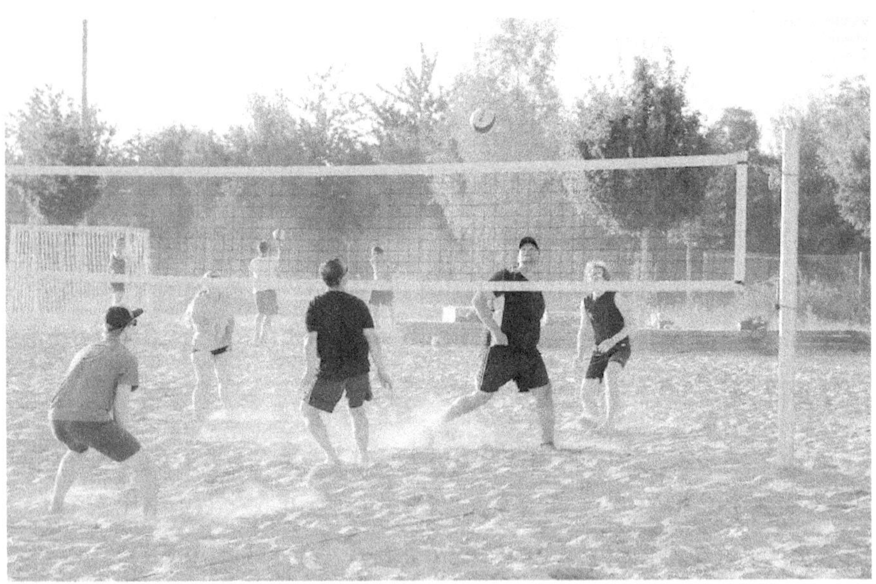

Chapter 1

Foundations of a Healthy Lifestyle

1. Understanding the Modern Health Crisis

In the 21st century, we find ourselves in the midst of a paradox. Despite unprecedented advancements in medical technology and a wealth of information at our fingertips, we are facing a global health crisis of staggering proportions. This crisis is not characterized by infectious diseases that plagued previous generations, but by chronic, lifestyle-related conditions that have become alarmingly common.

The statistics paint a grim picture. According to the World Health Organization, noncommunicable diseases (NCDs) such as heart disease, stroke, cancer, diabetes, and chronic lung disease are collectively responsible for almost 70% of all deaths worldwide. These diseases, once considered "diseases of affluence," now affect people of all socioeconomic backgrounds in both developed and developing countries.

Several factors contribute to this modern health crisis:

1. **Dietary shifts**: The global diet has undergone a dramatic transformation in recent decades. Processed foods high in sugar, salt, and unhealthy fats have replaced traditional, whole-food diets in many parts of the world. This nutritional transition has led to increased rates of obesity, diabetes, and cardiovascular diseases.

2. **Sedentary lifestyles**: Technological advancements, while improving many aspects of our lives, have also led to increasingly sedentary behaviors. From desk jobs to leisure activities centered around screens, physical inactivity has become the norm for many.

3. **Environmental factors**: Urbanization, pollution, and exposure to various chemicals in our environment have been linked to increased rates of certain cancers and respiratory diseases.

4. **Chronic stress**: The fast-paced nature of modern life, coupled with economic pressures and social expectations, has led to unprecedented levels of chronic stress, which is linked to a host of health problems.

5. **Sleep deprivation**: In our 24/7 society, sleep is often sacrificed in favor of work or leisure activities, leading to a host of health issues.

Understanding this crisis is the first step towards addressing it. By recognizing the root causes of our modern health challenges, we can begin to make informed decisions about our lifestyle choices and take control of our well-being.

2. The Impact of Sedentary Lifestyles

The human body is designed for movement, yet modern life often requires us to remain stationary for extended periods. This shift towards sedentary behavior has profound implications for our health.

Sedentary lifestyles are characterized by prolonged periods of sitting or lying down, with minimal physical activity. This includes time spent at desk jobs, commuting, watching television, or using computers and mobile devices for leisure. The consequences of such inactivity are far-reaching:

1. **Increased risk of chronic diseases**: Prolonged sitting has been linked to higher risks of heart disease, type 2 diabetes, and certain types of cancer. A study published in the Annals of Internal Medicine found that sitting for extended periods was associated with a higher risk of cardiovascular disease, cancer, and all-cause mortality.

2. **Musculoskeletal problems**: Lack of movement can lead to muscle weakness, poor posture, and chronic pain, particularly in the lower back, neck, and shoulders.

3. **Reduced metabolic function**: Sedentary behavior slows down metabolism, leading to decreased calorie burn and increased fat storage. This contributes to weight gain and obesity.

4.   **Impaired cognitive function**: Physical inactivity has been associated with reduced cognitive performance and an increased risk of depression and anxiety.

5.   **Decreased cardiovascular health**: A sedentary lifestyle can lead to poor circulation, increased blood pressure, and a higher risk of blood clots.

6.   **Weakened bones**: Lack of weight-bearing activity can lead to decreased bone density, increasing the risk of osteoporosis.

The insidious nature of sedentary behavior lies in its seeming innocuousness. Unlike smoking or excessive alcohol consumption, sitting doesn't feel harmful in the moment. However, its cumulative effects over time can be just as detrimental to health.

Recognizing the dangers of sedentary lifestyles is crucial for motivating change. In the following sections, we'll explore strategies for incorporating more movement into daily life and the numerous benefits of regular physical activity.

3. Importance of Physical Activity

Physical activity is a cornerstone of a healthy lifestyle, offering a myriad of benefits that extend far beyond mere weight management. Regular exercise is not just about sculpting the body; it's about optimizing overall health, enhancing quality of life, and preventing a wide array of diseases.

The benefits of regular physical activity include:

1. **Cardiovascular health**: Exercise strengthens the heart, improves circulation, and helps regulate blood pressure. This leads to a reduced risk of heart disease, stroke, and other cardiovascular problems.

2. **Weight management**: Physical activity burns calories and builds muscle, helping to maintain a healthy weight and body composition.

3. **Improved mental health**: Exercise releases endorphins, the body's natural mood elevators. Regular physical activity has been shown to reduce symptoms of depression and anxiety, improve self-esteem, and enhance overall mental well-being.

4. **Enhanced cognitive function**: Exercise increases blood flow to the brain, promoting the growth of new brain cells and improving memory and cognitive performance.

5. **Stronger bones and muscles**: Weight-bearing exercises and resistance training help build and maintain bone density, reducing the risk of osteoporosis. They also strengthen muscles, improving overall functionality and reducing the risk of injuries.

6. **Better sleep**: Regular physical activity can help you fall asleep faster and deepen your sleep, leading to more restorative rest.

7. **Increased energy levels**: Although it might seem counterintuitive, regular exercise actually boosts energy levels and reduces fatigue.

8. **Enhanced immune function**: Moderate, regular exercise has been shown to boost the immune system, potentially reducing the risk of infections and certain diseases.

9. **Improved balance and coordination**: Physical activity, especially as we age, helps maintain and improve balance and coordination, reducing the risk of falls.

10. **Increased longevity**: Studies have consistently shown that regular physical activity is associated with a longer life span and a reduced risk of premature death.

The World Health Organization recommends that adults aged 18-64 should do at least 150 minutes of moderate-intensity aerobic physical activity or at least 75 minutes of vigorous-intensity aerobic physical activity throughout the week. Additionally, muscle-strengthening activities should be done involving major muscle groups on 2 or more days a week.

It's important to note that these are minimum recommendations, and more activity generally provides greater health benefits. Moreover, any amount of physical activity is better than none. Even small increases in physical activity can have substantial health benefits, especially for those who are currently inactive.

In the context of our modern, often sedentary lifestyles, incorporating regular physical activity is not just beneficial—it's essential. Whether it's a structured exercise routine, active commuting, or simply taking regular breaks to move and stretch throughout the day, finding ways to increase physical activity is a crucial step towards better health.

4. Macronutrients: The Big Three

Proper nutrition and hydration are fundamental to good health, providing our bodies with the essential nutrients and fluids needed for optimal functioning. Understanding the basics of nutrition and staying adequately hydrated can significantly impact our overall well-being.

Nutrition

A balanced diet should include a variety of foods from all food groups to ensure you're getting all the necessary nutrients. Here are some key principles:

1. **Macronutrients**: These are the nutrients we need in larger quantities:

    o Carbohydrates: Provide energy and should come primarily from whole grains, fruits, and vegetables.

    o Proteins: Essential for building and repairing tissues. Sources include lean meats, fish, eggs, legumes, and dairy.

    o Fats: Necessary for hormone production and nutrient absorption. Focus on healthy fats from sources like nuts, seeds, avocados, and olive oil.

2. **Micronutrients**: These are needed in smaller amounts but are crucial for various bodily functions:

   o Vitamins: Essential for immune function, energy production, and overall health.

   o Minerals: Important for bone health, fluid balance, and many other bodily processes.

3. **Fiber**: Aids digestion promotes feelings of fullness, and supports gut health. Found in fruits, vegetables, whole grains, and legumes.

4. **Portion control**: Even healthy foods should be consumed in moderation. Understanding appropriate portion sizes is key to maintaining a healthy weight.

5. **Limit processed foods**: These often contain added sugars, unhealthy fats, and excessive salt, which can contribute to various health problems when consumed in large quantities.

6. **Eat a rainbow**: Consuming a variety of colorful fruits and vegetables ensures a wide range of nutrients and beneficial plant compounds.

Hydration

Water is essential for life, playing a crucial role in nearly every bodily function. Proper hydration:

1. **Regulates body temperature**

2. **Aids in digestion**

3. **Facilitates nutrient transport**

4. **Cushions joints**

5. **Removes waste products**

The often-cited recommendation is to drink 8 glasses (64 ounces) of water per day, but individual needs can vary based on factors like activity level, climate, and overall health. A good rule of thumb is to drink enough so that you rarely feel thirsty, and your urine is colorless or light yellow.

It's important to note that while water is the best choice for hydration, other beverages and water-rich foods can also contribute to your daily fluid intake. However, be mindful of drinks that contain caffeine or alcohol, as these can have a diuretic effect.

By focusing on a balanced diet rich in whole foods and staying properly hydrated, you create a strong foundation for overall health and well-being.

5. The Role of Sleep in Overall Health

Sleep is a fundamental biological process that is often overlooked in our fast-paced society. However, quality sleep is as essential to our health as proper nutrition and regular exercise. During sleep, our bodies undergo crucial processes of repair, regeneration, and consolidation of memories.

The importance of sleep extends to various aspects of our health:

1. **Physical Health:**

o Sleep is crucial for the repair and growth of tissues, including muscles and blood vessels.

- It plays a vital role in maintaining a healthy immune system.

- Adequate sleep is associated with better weight management and reduced risk of obesity.

- Chronic sleep deprivation has been linked to increased risks of heart disease, kidney disease, high blood pressure, and diabetes.

2. **Mental Health**:

- Sleep is essential for cognitive functions such as attention, learning, and memory consolidation.

- Lack of sleep can lead to mood disturbances, increased stress, and heightened risk of depression and anxiety.

- Chronic sleep deprivation can impair decision-making and increase the risk of accidents.

3. **Hormonal Balance**:

- Sleep regulates the production of various hormones, including growth hormone, which is crucial for cell repair and regeneration.

o It affects the balance of ghrelin and leptin, hormones that control hunger and fullness, which is why poor sleep is often associated with overeating and weight gain.

4. **Metabolic Health:**

o Adequate sleep helps maintain insulin sensitivity, reducing the risk of type 2 diabetes.

o It plays a role in regulating glucose metabolism and maintaining a healthy metabolism.

For optimal health, adults generally need between 7-9 hours of sleep per night. However, individual needs may vary. The quality of sleep is just as important as the quantity. Good sleep hygiene practices can help improve sleep quality:

- Maintain a consistent sleep schedule, even on weekends.

- Create a relaxing bedtime routine.

- Ensure your bedroom is dark, quiet, and cool.

- Avoid screens (phones, tablets, computers) for at least an hour before bed.

- Limit caffeine and alcohol consumption, especially in the evening.

- Regular exercise can improve sleep quality but avoid vigorous exercise close to bedtime.

In our 24/7 society, it's easy to sacrifice sleep for work or leisure activities. However, prioritizing sleep is a crucial investment in your health and well-being. By understanding the vital role of sleep and implementing good sleep habits, you can significantly improve your overall health and quality of life.

6. Stress Management Techniques

Stress is an inevitable part of modern life, but chronic, unmanaged stress can have severe implications for both physical and mental health. Learning effective stress management techniques is crucial for maintaining overall well-being and resilience in the face of life's challenges.

Here are some proven stress management techniques:

1. **Mindfulness and Meditation**:

   o Mindfulness involves focusing on the present moment without judgment.

   o Regular meditation practice can reduce stress, anxiety, and depression.

   o Even a few minutes of mindfulness daily can make a significant difference.

2. **Deep Breathing Exercises**:

o Controlled breathing can activate the body's relaxation response.

- o Try the 4-7-8 technique: Inhale for 4 seconds, hold for 7, exhale for 8.

- o Practice deep breathing regularly, not just in stressful moments.

3. **Regular Physical Exercise**:

- o Exercise releases endorphins, natural mood elevators.

- o It can also serve as a form of moving meditation, helping to clear the mind.

- o Aim for at least 30 minutes of moderate exercise most days of the week.

4. **Time Management and Prioritization**:

- o Learn to prioritize tasks and say no to non-essential commitments.

- o Use tools like calendars and to-do lists to stay organized.

- o Break large tasks into smaller, manageable steps.

5. **Social Connections**:

- o Maintain strong social connections with friends and family.

- o Talking about your stress with trusted individuals can provide relief and perspective.

  - o Don't hesitate to seek professional help when needed.

6. **Healthy Sleep Habits**:

  - o Prioritize getting 7-9 hours of quality sleep each night.

  - o Establish a consistent sleep schedule and relaxing bedtime routine.

7. **Nutrition**:

  - o A balanced diet can help your body cope with stress.

  - o Limit caffeine and alcohol, which can exacerbate stress and anxiety.

  - o Stay hydrated, as dehydration can increase stress hormones.

8. **Hobbies and Leisure Activities**:

  - o Engage in activities you enjoy taking your mind off stressors.

  - o Creative pursuits like art, music, or writing can be particularly therapeutic.

9. **Nature Exposure**:

- o Spending time in nature has been shown to reduce stress and improve mood.

    - o Even looking at images of nature or having plants in your workspace can help.

10. **Progressive Muscle Relaxation**:

    - o This technique involves tensing and then relaxing different muscle groups.

    - o It can help reduce physical tension associated with stress.

11. **Cognitive Restructuring**:

    - o Learn to identify and challenge negative thought patterns.

    - o Reframe stressful situations in a more balanced, realistic way.

12. **Limit Information Overload**:

    - o Set boundaries on news consumption and social media use.

    - o Create tech-free zones or times in your day.

Remember, stress management is highly individual. What works for one person may not work for another. It's important to experiment with different techniques and find what resonates with you. Also, consistency is key – incorporate these practices into your daily routine for the best results.

By actively managing stress, you not only improve your mental well-being but also support your overall physical health. Chronic stress can contribute to a host of health problems, including heart disease, digestive issues, and weakened immune function. Therefore, effective stress management is a crucial component of a healthy lifestyle.

In conclusion, the foundations of a healthy lifestyle are multifaceted, encompassing physical activity, proper nutrition and hydration, adequate sleep, and effective stress management. By understanding and addressing each of these areas, you can create a solid base for overall health and well-being. Remember, small, consistent changes can lead to significant improvements over time.

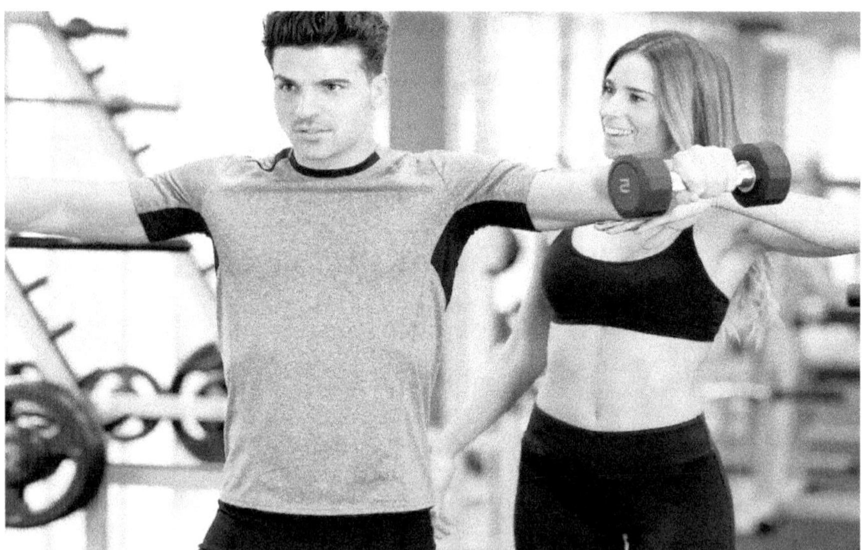

The journey to better health is ongoing, but with these foundational principles in place, you're well-equipped to navigate the path to a healthier, more vibrant life.

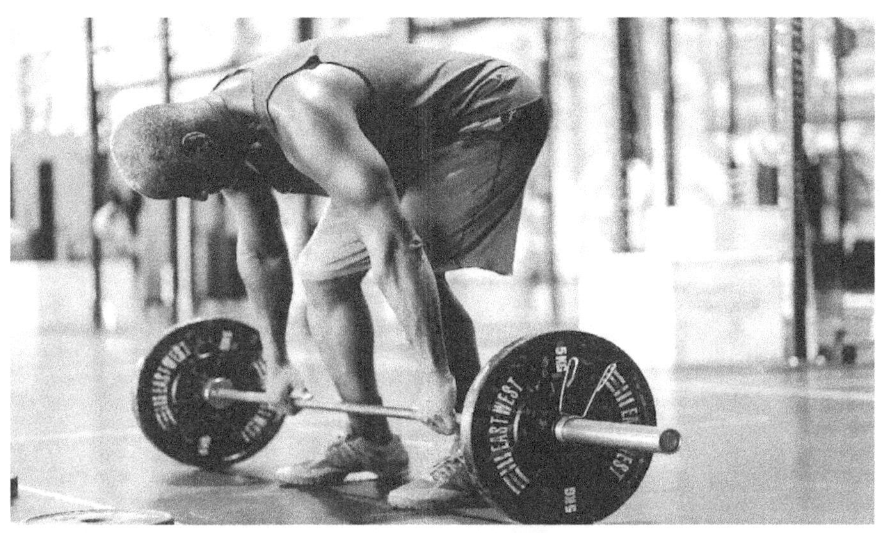

Chapter 2

Essential Principles of Health and Fitness

1. Defining True Fitness

When you hear the word "fitness," what comes to mind? For many people, it might be images of muscular athletes, marathon runners, or perfectly toned Instagram models. But true fitness is about so much more than how you look or how far you can run. It's about feeling good, being healthy, and having the energy to enjoy life to its fullest.

Think of fitness as your body's way of saying, "I'm ready for anything!" It's not just about being able to lift heavy weights or run long distances. It's about being able to play with your kids without getting tired, climb a flight of stairs without getting out of breath, or dance all night at a party. It's about waking up in the morning feeling refreshed and energized, ready to tackle whatever the day might bring.

True fitness is a balance of physical and mental well-being. It's about:

o Having a strong, healthy body that can handle daily tasks with ease

o Feeling confident and comfortable in your own skin

o Having plenty of energy to do the things you love

o Being able to handle stress without feeling overwhelmed

o Sleeping well and waking up refreshed

o Enjoying a variety of foods without guilt or restriction

o Being able to participate in fun activities and sports

o Feeling positive and optimistic about life

Remember, fitness looks different for everyone. A professional athlete's idea of fitness might be very different from a busy parent's or a retiree's. The key is finding what fitness means for you and working towards that in a way that makes you feel good.

In the next sections, we'll explore the different components of fitness and how they all work together to create a healthier, happier you. But always keep in mind that true fitness is about improving your own health and well-being, not comparing yourself to others or trying to meet unrealistic standards. It's a personal journey, and every small step you take is a victory worth celebrating!

2. The Five Components of Fitness

Just like a car needs different parts to run smoothly, our bodies need different types of fitness to function at their best. These are called the five components of fitness. Think of them as the ingredients in your fitness recipe. When you mix them all together in the right way, you get a healthier, stronger, more flexible you!

Let's break down each component and see why it's important:

a. Aerobic Endurance

Aerobic endurance is all about how long your body can keep moving. It's like your body's battery life. The better your aerobic endurance, the longer you can do activities without getting tired.

Imagine you're playing tag with your friends. If you have good aerobic endurance, you can run around for a long time without needing to stop and catch your breath. Or think about climbing several flights of stairs – with good aerobic endurance, you can reach the top without feeling like you just ran a marathon!

Activities that help improve aerobic endurance include:

- Running or jogging
- Swimming
- Cycling
- Dancing
- Jumping rope
- Brisk walking

Why is it important? Good aerobic endurance helps your heart and lungs work better. It gives you more energy for daily activities and helps you recover faster when you do get tired.

b. Muscular Strength

Muscular strength is about how much force your muscles can produce. It's like your body's power level. The stronger your muscles, the more you can lift, push, or pull.

Think about opening a tight jar lid or carrying heavy grocery bags. That's muscular strength in action! It's not just about being able to lift weights at the gym (although that's one way to build strength). It's about making everyday tasks easier.

Activities that help improve muscular strength include:

- Weight lifting

- Push-ups

- Pull-ups

- Using resistance bands

- Rock climbing

- Carrying heavy objects (safely!)

Why is it important? Good muscular strength makes daily tasks easier. It helps protect your joints from injury, improves your posture, and can even boost your metabolism.

c. Muscular Endurance

Muscular endurance is about how long your muscles can keep working without getting tired. It's like your muscles' stamina. The better your muscular endurance, the longer you can do repetitive activities without your muscles giving up.

Imagine you're helping paint a wall or raking leaves in the yard. These activities require you to repeat the same motions over and over. Good muscular endurance helps you keep going without your arms feeling like jelly!

Activities that help improve muscular endurance include:

- Doing many repetitions with lighter weights
- Planks and wall sits
- Swimming
- Rowing
- Cycling
- Body weight exercises like squats or push-ups

Why is it important? Good muscular endurance helps you perform repetitive tasks without getting tired quickly. It's great for sports, household chores, and many jobs that require repeated physical actions.

d. Flexibility

Flexibility is about how well you can move and stretch your body. It's like being a human rubber band! The more flexible you are, the easier it is to bend, reach, and move in different directions.

Think about trying to touch your toes or reaching for something on a high shelf. That's flexibility in action. It's not about being able to do the splits (unless you want to!). It's about being able to move freely and comfortably in your daily life.

Activities that help improve flexibility include:

- Stretching exercises

- Yoga

- Pilates

- Dancing

- Tai Chi

- Even simple activities like reaching for your toes or doing arm circles

Why is it important? Good flexibility helps prevent injuries, reduces muscle soreness, improves posture, and makes it easier to do a wide range of activities. It can also help you feel more relaxed and less tense.

e. Body Composition

Body composition is about the balance of fat, muscle, bone, and other tissues in your body. It's like your body's building blocks. Having a healthy body composition means having the right amount of each component for your individual needs.

It's important to note that body composition is not about being skinny or looking a certain way. Two people can weigh the same but have very different body compositions. For example, muscle is denser than fat, so someone with more muscle might weigh more but look leaner.

Activities that help improve body composition include:

- A combination of aerobic exercise and strength training

- Eating a balanced, nutritious diet

- Getting enough sleep

- Managing stress

Why is it important? A healthy body composition reduces your risk of certain health problems, gives you more energy, and can help you feel more confident and comfortable in your body.

Remember, all five of these components work together to create overall fitness. It's not about being perfect in all areas, but about finding a balance that works for you and your lifestyle. In the next sections, we'll explore how your mind plays a role in fitness and how to set goals that work for you.

3. The Mind-Body Connection in Fitness

Have you ever noticed how your mood can affect how you feel physically? Or how exercise can make you feel happier? That's the mind-body connection in action! Our minds and bodies are not separate – they're deeply connected and constantly influencing each other.

When it comes to fitness, this connection is super important. Here's why:

1. **Motivation**: Your mind is what gets you moving in the first place. If you're feeling positive and motivated, you're more likely to want to exercise and eat healthy foods.

2. **Stress Management**: Exercise is a great way to reduce stress. When you're stressed, your body releases hormones that can make you feel tense and anxious. Physical activity helps burn off these stress hormones, making you feel more relaxed.

3. **Body Awareness**: Being in tune with your body helps you know when to push harder and when to rest. This awareness can help prevent injuries and make your workouts more effective.

4. **Confidence**: As you get fitter and achieve your goals, your confidence grows. This positive mindset can motivate you to keep going and try new things.

5. **Focus**: Many forms of exercise, like running or yoga, can help improve your concentration and focus. This can benefit other areas of your life too, like work or school.

6. **Emotional Release**: Physical activity can be a great way to release emotions. Had a frustrating day? A good workout can help you let it all out and feel better.

7. **Mindfulness**: Activities like yoga and tai chi combine physical movement with mindfulness, helping you stay present and reduce worries about the past or future.

8. **Sleep**: Regular exercise can help improve your sleep quality, which in turn helps your body recover and your mind stay sharp.

So, how can you strengthen this mind-body connection? Here are a few ideas:

- o **Practice mindfulness**: Pay attention to how your body feels during different activities. Notice your breathing, how your muscles feel, and your energy levels.

- o **Set intentions**: Before you work out, take a moment to think about why you're doing it. Is it to feel stronger? To reduce stress? To have fun? Setting an intention can make your workout more meaningful.

- o **Use positive self-talk**: Encourage yourself like you would a good friend. Instead of "I can't do this," try "I'm getting stronger every day."

- o **Try mind-body exercises**: Activities like yoga, Pilates, or tai chi are great for connecting your mind and body.

- o **Celebrate small victories**: Notice and appreciate the little improvements. Maybe you can hold a plank for a few seconds longer or you feel less out of breath climbing stairs.

Remember, fitness isn't just about your body – it's about your whole self. By nurturing the connection between your mind and body, you can create a more balanced, enjoyable approach to fitness that benefits all aspects of your life.

4. Setting Realistic Fitness Goals

Setting goals is like planning a road trip. You need to know where you're going and how you're going to get there. But when it comes to fitness goals, it's important to make sure your destination is somewhere you can actually reach!

Here's how to set realistic fitness goals that will keep you motivated and moving forward:

1. **Start Where You Are**: Before setting goals, take an honest look at your current fitness level. If you haven't exercised in years, running a marathon next month probably isn't realistic. But walking for 15 minutes a day might be a great place to start.

2. **Make Your Goals Specific**: Instead of saying "I want to get fit," try something like "I want to be able to jog for 20 minutes without stopping." Specific goals are easier to plan for and achieve.

3. **Make Your Goals Measurable**: How will you know when you've reached your goal? For example, "I want to do 10 push-ups" is measurable. You can track your progress and know exactly when you've succeeded.

4. **Set Short-Term and Long-Term Goals**: Having a big, exciting long-term goal is great, but it can feel overwhelming. Break it down into smaller, short-term goals. If your long-term goal is to run a 5K, your short-term goals might be to run for 5 minutes without stopping, then 10 minutes, and so on.

5. **Be Realistic**: It's great to challenge yourself, but make sure your goals are achievable. If you set impossible goals, you'll just end up frustrated. Remember, small improvements add up to big changes over time!

6. **Set a Timeframe**: Decide when you want to achieve your goal. This helps you stay focused and gives you a way to plan your progress. But be flexible – if you need more time, that's okay!

7. **Focus on Actions, Not Just Outcomes**: While it's great to have a goal like "lose 10 pounds," it's even better to focus on the actions that will get you there, like "exercise for 30 minutes, 3 times a week" or "eat 5 servings of vegetables every day."

8. **Write Your Goals Down**: Put your goals somewhere you can see them regularly. This helps keep you focused and motivated.

9. **Share Your Goals**: Tell a friend or family member about your goals. They can offer support and encouragement, and knowing someone else knows about your goals can help keep you accountable.

10. **Celebrate Your Progress**: Don't wait until you've reached your final goal to celebrate. Acknowledge each small victory along the way. This helps keep you motivated and makes the journey more enjoyable.

Remember, your fitness journey is personal. Your goals should reflect what's important to you, not what someone else thinks you should do. Maybe your goal is to have more energy to play with your kids, or to feel more confident in your body, or to be able to hike to the top of a mountain. Whatever your goals are, make sure they're meaningful to you.

And don't forget – it's okay to adjust your goals as you go along. As you learn more about yourself and what you're capable of, you might find that you want to aim higher, or that you need to take things a bit slower. That's all part of the journey!

5. The Importance of Consistency and Patience

Imagine you're planting a garden. You wouldn't plant a seed and expect to see a full-grown plant the next day, would you? Growing a garden takes time, regular care, and patience. The same is true for your fitness journey. Consistency and patience are like the water and sunlight that help your fitness "garden" grow.

Let's break down why these two qualities are so important:

Consistency: The Key to Progress

Consistency means doing something regularly, even when you don't feel like it. Here's why it's so crucial:

1. **Builds Habits**: When you do something consistently, it becomes a habit. Over time, exercise becomes a natural part of your routine, like brushing your teeth.

2. **Steady Progress**: Consistent effort leads to steady progress. It might be slow, but it adds up over time. Remember, slow progress is still progress!

3. **Prevents Setbacks**: Regular exercise helps maintain your fitness level. If you exercise sporadically, you might find yourself starting from scratch each time.

4. **Boosts Motivation**: As you see the results of your consistent efforts, you'll feel more motivated to keep going.

5. **Improves Overall Health**: Regular exercise has cumulative benefits for your health, like improving your heart health, strengthening your bones, and boosting your immune system.

Tips for staying consistent:

- Start small: It's better to do a little bit every day than to overdo it and burn out.

- Schedule your workouts: Treat them like important appointments.

- Find activities you enjoy: You're more likely to stick with something you like doing.

- Be flexible: If you can't do your planned workout, do something else instead. A short walk is better than nothing!

Patience: The Art of Trusting the Process

Patience means understanding that good things take time. Here's why patience is so important in your fitness journey:

1. **Prevents Frustration**: When you're patient, you're less likely to get discouraged if you don't see immediate results.

2. **Allows for Real Change**: Lasting changes in your body and health take time. Patience allows these changes to happen naturally.

3. **Reduces Risk of Injury**: Being patient means you're more likely to progress at a safe pace, reducing the risk of overdoing it and getting hurt.

4. **Encourages Long-Term Thinking**: Patience helps you focus on long-term health and fitness, not just quick fixes.

5. **Builds Mental Toughness**: Learning to be patient is a valuable skill that can help in all areas of life, not just fitness.

Tips for cultivating patience:

- Focus on the process, not just the end goal.

- Celebrate small victories along the way.

- Keep a journal to track your progress over time.

- Remember that everyone's journey is different – don't compare yourself to others.

Consistency and Patience Working Together

Consistency and patience are like best friends – they work best when they're together. Here's how:

- Consistent effort + patience = lasting results

- Consistency gives you data points to track your progress, while patience gives you the time to see the bigger picture.

- Being consistent shows you're committed, while being patient shows you understand that real change takes time.

Remember, your fitness journey is a marathon, not a sprint. There will be ups and downs, fast progress and slow progress. But if you stay consistent and patient, you'll be amazed at how far you can go.

Think back to our garden analogy. Some days you might not see any change in your plants. But under the surface, roots are growing stronger. Your fitness is the same way. Even on days when you don't see or feel a difference, your consistent efforts are making you stronger and healthier.

So keep showing up, keep putting in the effort, and be patient with yourself. Your future self will thank you for the consistent care you're putting in today. Remember, the best time to plant a tree was 20 years ago. The second best time is now. So start where you are, use what you have, and do what you can. With consistency and patience, you'll be amazed at how your fitness "garden" will grow!

6. The Importance of Consistency and Patience

When it comes to fitness, consistency and patience are like your secret weapons. They might not be as exciting as trying the latest workout trend, but they're the key to real, lasting results. Let's break down why these two qualities are so crucial:

Consistency: The Foundation of Progress

Consistency means sticking to your fitness plan regularly, even when you don't feel like it. Here's why it's so important:

1. **Builds Habits**: When you exercise consistently, it becomes a habit, like brushing your teeth. It starts to feel weird if you don't do it!

2. **Steady Progress**: Small, consistent efforts add up over time. It's like saving money - a little bit each day can turn into a lot over a year.

3. **Prevents Setbacks**: Regular exercise helps maintain your fitness level. If you exercise sporadically, you might find yourself starting from scratch each time.

4. **Hormonal Benefits**: Consistent exercise helps regulate hormones that affect your mood, sleep, and overall health.

5. **Builds Momentum**: The more consistent you are, the more you'll want to keep going. Success breeds success!

Tips for staying consistent:

- Start small: It's better to do a little bit every day than to overdo it and burn out.

- Schedule your workouts: Treat them like important appointments.

- Find activities you enjoy: You're more likely to stick with something you like doing.

- Be flexible: If you can't do your planned workout, do something else instead. A short walk is better than nothing!

Patience: The Key to Long-Term Success

Patience means understanding that good things take time. Here's why patience is crucial in your fitness journey:

1. **Allows for Real Change**: Your body needs time to adapt to new exercise routines. Patience gives your body the time it needs to get stronger and fitter.

2. **Prevents Burnout**: Trying to do too much too soon can lead to exhaustion or injury. Patience helps you progress at a sustainable pace.

3. **Builds Lasting Habits**: Quick fixes rarely last. Patience allows you to build habits that stick with you for life.

4. **Reduces Frustration**: When you're patient, you're less likely to get discouraged if you don't see immediate results.

5. **Encourages Long-Term Thinking**: Patience helps you focus on long-term health and fitness, not just quick fixes.

Tips for cultivating patience:

- Set realistic goals: Understand that significant changes take time.

- Track your progress: Look for small improvements - they add up!

- Celebrate non-scale victories: Notice improvements in your energy, mood, or how your clothes fit.

- Remember why you started: Focus on your overall health and well-being, not just quick results.

Consistency and Patience Working Together

Consistency and patience are like best friends - they work best when they're together. Here's how:

- Consistent effort + patience = lasting results

- Consistency gives you data points to track your progress, while patience gives you the time to see the bigger picture.

- Being consistent shows you're committed, while being patient shows you understand that real change takes time.

Remember, your fitness journey is a marathon, not a sprint. There will be ups and downs, fast progress and slow progress. But if you stay consistent and patient, you'll be amazed at how far you can go.

Think of it like growing a plant. You need to water it consistently (that's your regular exercise and healthy habits), but you also need to be patient and give it time to grow. You wouldn't dig up a seed every day to see if it's growing, right? The same goes for your fitness - trust the process, stay consistent, and be patient. Before you know it, you'll see the results of your hard work blooming!

7. Adapting Your Fitness Plan as You Progress

As you continue on your fitness journey, you'll notice changes in your body and abilities. What was once challenging might become easy, and you might find yourself ready for new goals. This is where adapting your fitness plan comes in. It's all about making adjustments to keep challenging yourself and moving forward.

Why Adaptation is Important

1. **Prevents Plateaus**: Your body is amazingly adaptable. If you do the same workout all the time, your body gets used to it and you stop seeing progress. Changing things up keeps your body guessing and improving.

2. **Maintains Interest**: Doing the same thing all the time can get boring. Mixing things up keeps your workouts interesting and fun.

3. **Allows for Goal Progression**: As you achieve your initial fitness goals, you'll want to set new ones. Your fitness plan should evolve to match your new aspirations.

4. **Reduces Risk of Overuse Injuries**: Doing the same movements repeatedly can sometimes lead to overuse injuries. Varying your routine can help prevent this.

How to Adapt Your Fitness Plan

1. **Gradually Increase Intensity**: This could mean lifting heavier weights, running faster or farther, or doing more repetitions of an exercise.

2. **Change Your Routine**: Try new exercises or activities. If you usually run, maybe try cycling or swimming for a change.

3. **Adjust Your Frequency**: You might find you're ready to add an extra workout day to your week.

4. **Modify Your Duration**: As your endurance improves, you might be able to exercise for longer periods.

5. **Play with Rest Periods**: Shortening the rest time between sets can increase the intensity of your workout.

6. **Try New Techniques**: Things like supersets, circuit training, or interval training can add new challenges to your routine.

7. **Reassess Your Nutrition**: As your activity level changes, your nutritional needs might change too.

Signs It's Time to Adapt Your Plan

1. **You're No Longer Challenged**: If your workouts feel too easy, it's time to step it up.

2. **You're Not Seeing Progress**: If you've stopped seeing improvements in your strength, endurance, or other goals, you might need to change things up.

3. **You're Bored**: If you're dreading your workouts because they're monotonous, it's definitely time for a change.

4. **You've Reached Your Initial Goals**: Celebrate, then set new goals!

5. **Your Schedule Has Changed**: Life happens. If your current plan no longer fits your schedule, adapt it so you can stay consistent.

Tips for Successful Adaptation

1. **Make Gradual Changes**: Don't overhaul your entire routine at once. Small, progressive changes are more sustainable.

2. **Listen to Your Body**: Push yourself, but not to the point of pain or exhaustion.

3. **Keep Track of Your Progress**: This will help you see when it's time to make changes and what changes are effective.

4. **Be Patient**: Give each change a few weeks to see how your body responds before making more adjustments.

5. **Seek Guidance if Needed**: If you're not sure how to progress, consider working with a fitness professional who can guide you.

Remember, adapting your fitness plan isn't about constantly changing everything. It's about making smart, gradual adjustments to keep you moving towards your goals. Your fitness journey is uniquely yours, and your plan should reflect that. Embrace the process of learning about your body and what works best for you. With consistency, patience, and smart adaptation, you'll continue to grow stronger, fitter, and healthier!

Wrap up: Your Fitness Journey Starts Now

We've covered a lot of ground in this chapter, exploring the essential principles of health and fitness. From understanding what true fitness means, to breaking down the five components of fitness, to recognizing the importance of the mind-body connection, setting realistic goals, and understanding the crucial roles of consistency, patience, and adaptation.

Remember, fitness is not a destination, but a journey. It's not about reaching a certain weight or being able to lift a specific amount. It's about feeling good in your body, having the energy to enjoy life, and taking care of your health for the long term.

Here are some key takeaways to keep in mind as you move forward on your fitness journey:

1. **True fitness is holistic**: It's not just about how you look, but how you feel, both physically and mentally.

2. **Balance is key**: Aim to improve all five components of fitness - aerobic endurance, muscular strength, muscular endurance, flexibility, and body composition.

3. **Your mind matters**: Don't underestimate the power of the mind-body connection in your fitness journey.

4. **Set SMART goals**: Make your fitness goals Specific, Measurable, Achievable, Relevant, and Time-bound.

5. **Consistency is crucial**: Regular, consistent effort is more important than sporadic intense workouts.

6. **Be patient**: Real, lasting changes take time. Trust the process and keep going.

7. **Adapt and grow**: Be ready to adjust your fitness plan as you progress and your goals evolve.

8. **Enjoy the journey**: Find activities you enjoy. Fitness should enhance your life, not feel like a punishment.

9. **Everyone is different**: What works for someone else might not work for you, and that's okay. Your fitness journey is uniquely yours.

10. **Start where you are**: You don't need to be fit to start getting fit. Every journey begins with a single step.

As you embark on or continue your fitness journey, remember to be kind to yourself. There will be ups and downs, progress and setbacks. That's all part of the process. What matters most is that you keep moving forward, one step at a time.

Your future self will thank you for every healthy choice you make today. So why not start now? Choose one small thing you can do today to move towards your fitness goals. Maybe it's going for a 10-minute walk, doing some stretches, or planning some healthy meals for the week ahead. Whatever it is, take that step. Your journey to better health and fitness starts right here, right now.

Remember, you've got this! Here's to your health, your fitness, and your best life ahead. Let's get moving!

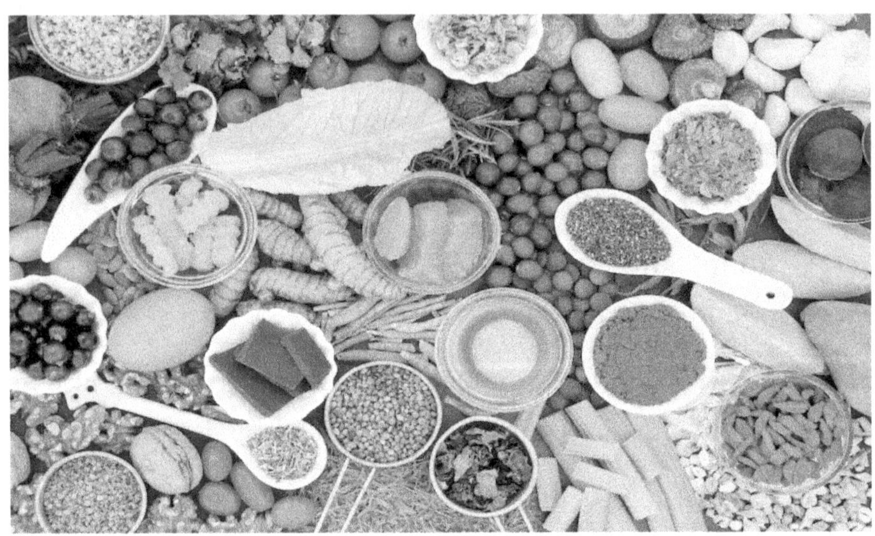

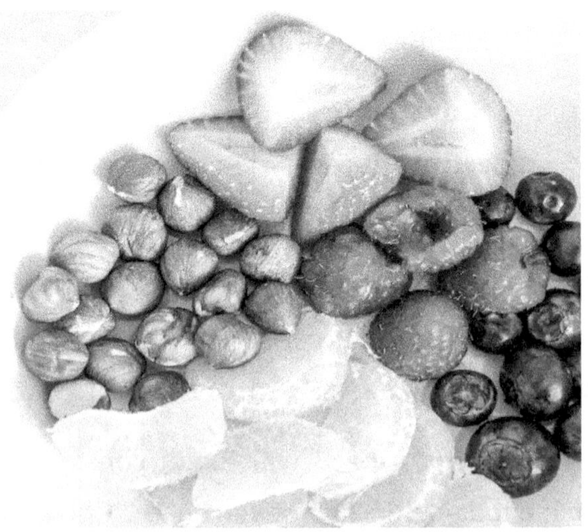

Chapter 3

Nutrition Fundamentals for Optimal Health

1. Understanding Macronutrients and Micronutrients

Imagine your body is like a fantastic machine. To keep it running smoothly, you need to give it the right fuel. That's where nutrients come in! There are two main types of nutrients your body needs: macronutrients and micronutrients. Let's explore what these are and why they're so important.

Macronutrients: The Big Three

Macronutrients are the nutrients your body needs in large amounts. There are three types of macronutrients:

1. **Carbohydrates**: These are your body's main source of energy. Think of carbs as the gasoline that keeps your body's engine running. They come in two main types:

     o   Simple carbs: Found in fruits, milk, and sugary foods. They give you quick energy.

o   Complex carbs: Found in whole grains, vegetables, and legumes. They provide longer-lasting energy.

Good sources of healthy carbs include whole grain bread, brown rice, fruits, vegetables, and beans.

2.   **Proteins**: Proteins are the building blocks of your body. They help build and repair tissues, make enzymes and hormones, and support your immune system. It's like the bricks and mortar that keep your body's structure strong. Good sources of protein include lean meats, fish, eggs, dairy products, beans, and nuts.

3.   **Fats**: Don't be scared of fats! Your body needs some fat to function properly. Fats help your body absorb certain vitamins, provide energy, and support cell growth. Think of fats as the oil that keeps your body's machine running smoothly. Healthy fats can be found in avocados, nuts, seeds, olive oil, and fatty fish like salmon.

Micronutrients: Small but Mighty

Micronutrients are nutrients your body needs in smaller amounts, but they're just as important! There are two main types:

1.   **Vitamins**: These are essential for various bodily functions, like boosting your immune system, helping your body heal, and supporting your metabolism. There are many different vitamins, each with its own special job. For example:

o   Vitamin C helps your immune system and helps your body absorb iron.

- o   Vitamin D helps your body absorb calcium for strong bones.

   - o   B vitamins help your body turn food into energy.

2. **Minerals**: These are important for things like strong bones, healthy blood, and balancing fluids in your body. Some important minerals include:

   - o   Calcium for strong bones and teeth.

   - o   Iron for healthy blood.

   - o   Potassium for heart health and muscle function.

You can get most of the micronutrients you need by eating a variety of colorful fruits and vegetables, whole grains, lean proteins, and dairy or dairy alternatives.

Why Balance Matters

Your body needs all of these nutrients to function at its best. It's like a symphony orchestra - each instrument (or nutrient) plays an important part, and when they all work together in the right balance, the result is beautiful music (or in this case, good health!).

Eating a variety of foods from all food groups helps ensure you're getting a good balance of all these important nutrients. In the next section, we'll talk more about how to create a balanced diet that supports your fitness goals.

Remember, good nutrition isn't about being perfect or never enjoying treats. It's about making informed choices most of the time and finding a balance that works for you. Small, consistent changes in your eating habits can lead to big improvements in your health and fitness over time!

2. The Role of Balanced Diet in Fitness

Now that we understand the different types of nutrients our bodies need, let's talk about how to put it all together. A balanced diet is like a superhero team for your body - each nutrient has its own special power, and when they work together, they help you feel and perform your best!

Why is a Balanced Diet Important for Fitness?

1. **Energy for Exercise**: The right balance of nutrients gives you the energy you need to work out and stay active throughout the day. Carbohydrates are especially important for fueling exercise.

2. **Muscle Building and Repair**: Protein is crucial for building and repairing muscles after exercise. It's like the construction crew that helps your muscles grow stronger.

3. **Recovery**: A balanced diet with plenty of vitamins and minerals helps your body recover faster after workouts. This means less soreness and more energy for your next session!

4. **Immune System Support**: Good nutrition keeps your immune system strong, which means you're less likely to get sick and miss workouts.

5. **Weight Management**: Whether your goal is to lose weight, gain muscle, or maintain your current weight, a balanced diet is key.

6. **Overall Health**: A balanced diet supports not just your fitness goals, but your overall health. This includes heart health, bone strength, digestive health, and even mental well-being.

What Does a Balanced Diet Look Like?

A balanced diet includes foods from all major food groups in the right proportions. Here's a simple way to think about it:

- **Fill half your plate with fruits and vegetables**: These provide essential vitamins, minerals, and fiber. Aim for a variety of colors to get different nutrients.

- **Make a quarter of your plate whole grains**: Things like brown rice, whole wheat bread, or oatmeal. These provide energy and fiber.

- **Make a quarter of your plate lean protein** : This could be chicken, fish, beans, tofu, or lean meat. Protein is crucial for muscle health.

- **Include some healthy fats**: Things like avocado, nuts, seeds, or olive oil. A little goes a long way!

- **Don't forget dairy or dairy alternatives**: These provide calcium and protein. If you don't eat dairy, look for fortified plant-based alternatives.

Tips for Maintaining a Balanced Diet

1. **Eat the Rainbow**: Different colored fruits and vegetables provide different nutrients. Try to include a variety of colors in your diet.

2. **Plan Ahead**: Planning your meals can help you ensure you're getting a good balance of nutrients throughout the day.

3. **Listen to Your Body**: Pay attention to how different foods make you feel. Everyone's needs are a bit different.

4. **Stay Hydrated**: Water is an essential part of a balanced diet. We'll talk more about hydration later in this chapter.

5. **Everything in Moderation**: It's okay to enjoy treats sometimes. The key is balance and moderation.

6. **Timing Matters**: Try to eat regularly throughout the day to keep your energy levels stable.

Remember, a balanced diet doesn't have to be complicated or restrictive. It's about making choices that nourish your body and support your fitness goals. In the next section, we'll talk about how to plan your meals to support your specific fitness goals.

3. Meal Planning for Fitness Goals

Meal planning is like creating a roadmap for your nutrition journey. It helps you stay on track with your fitness goals, saves time and money, and takes the guesswork out of "What should I eat?" Let's explore how to plan your meals based on different fitness goals.

General Tips for Meal Planning

Regardless of your specific goal, these tips can help make meal planning easier:

1. **Plan Weekly**: Take some time each week to plan your meals.

2. **Make a Grocery List**: This helps you stick to your plan and avoid impulse buys.

3. **Prep in Advance**: Washing and chopping veggies or cooking grains in advance can save time during the week.

4. **Use Leftovers Wisely**: Cook extra at dinner to use for lunch the next day.

5. **Keep It Simple**: You don't need to cook gourmet meals every day. Simple, nutritious meals work great!

Meal Planning for Different Fitness Goals

Goal: Weight Loss

If you're aiming to lose weight, focus on creating a slight calorie deficit while still getting all the nutrients you need.

- **Emphasize Vegetables**: They're low in calories but high in nutrients and fiber, which helps you feel full.

- **Include Lean Proteins**: These help you feel satisfied and support muscle maintenance.

- **Control Portions**: Use smaller plates and measure foods if needed.

- **Plan for Snacks**: Having healthy snacks on hand can prevent overeating later.

Sample Day:

- Breakfast: Oatmeal with berries and a sprinkle of nuts

- Snack: Apple slices with a small amount of peanut butter

- Lunch: Large salad with grilled chicken, lots of veggies, and a light dressing

- Snack: Carrot sticks with hummus

- Dinner: Baked fish with roasted vegetables and a small portion of brown rice

Goal: Muscle Gain

To build muscle, you need to eat enough calories to support growth, with an emphasis on protein.

- **Increase Protein Intake**: Aim for protein at every meal and snack.

- **Don't Skimp on Carbs**: You need carbs to fuel your workouts and support muscle growth.

- **Include Healthy Fats**: They help with hormone production, which is important for muscle growth.

Sample Day:

- Breakfast: Scrambled eggs with whole grain toast and avocado

- Snack: Greek yogurt with granola and fruit

- Lunch: Chicken breast with sweet potato and steamed broccoli

- Snack: Protein shake with banana

- Dinner: Lean beef stir fry with mixed vegetables and brown rice

Goal: Improve Athletic Performance

For better athletic performance, focus on balanced meals with a good mix of carbs for energy and protein for recovery.

- **Time Your Meals**: Eat a balanced meal 2-3 hours before exercise, and refuel within 30 minutes after.

- **Stay Hydrated**: We'll cover this more in the next section!

- **Include a Variety of Fruits and Vegetables**: These provide important vitamins and minerals for performance and recovery.

Sample Day:

- Breakfast: Whole grain cereal with milk, sliced banana, and a handful of nuts

- Pre-workout Snack: Apple with string cheese

- Lunch: Turkey and avocado sandwich on whole grain bread with a side of cherry tomatoes

- Post-workout: Chocolate milk (great for recovery!)

- Dinner: Grilled salmon with quinoa and roasted vegetables

Goal: Maintain Current Weight and Improve Overall Health

If you're happy with your current weight and just want to eat for general health and fitness, focus on balance and variety.

- **Follow the Balanced Plate Model**: Half vegetables, quarter protein, quarter whole grains.

- **Include a Variety of Foods**: This ensures you're getting a wide range of nutrients.

- **Listen to Your Hunger Cues**: Eat when you're hungry, stop when you're satisfied.

Sample Day:

- Breakfast: Yogurt parfait with granola, mixed berries, and a drizzle of honey

- Snack: Handful of mixed nuts

- Lunch: Lentil soup with a mixed green salad and a piece of fruit

- Snack: Whole grain crackers with cheese

- Dinner: Stir-fried tofu and vegetables with brown rice

Remember, these are just examples. Your specific needs may vary based on your body, activity level, and personal preferences. It's always a good idea to consult with a registered dietitian or your healthcare provider for personalized advice.

The key to successful meal planning is finding an approach that works for you and your lifestyle. Don't be afraid to experiment and adjust as you go along. With practice, you'll find a routine that supports your fitness goals and fits into your life!

4. Hydration Strategies

Water is like the oil in your car's engine – it keeps everything running smoothly. Staying properly hydrated is crucial for your overall health and fitness performance. Let's dive into why hydration is so important and how you can make sure you're getting enough fluids.

Why is Hydration Important?

1. **Regulates Body Temperature**: When you exercise, your body sweats to cool down. Proper hydration helps this process work efficiently.

2. **Supports Nutrient Transport**: Water helps carry nutrients to your cells and removes waste products.

3. **Lubricates Joints**: Staying hydrated helps keep your joints cushioned and moving smoothly.

4. **Boosts Energy**: Even mild dehydration can make you feel tired and less motivated to exercise.

5. **Improves Performance**: Good hydration can help you perform better during workouts and competitions.

6. **Aids Digestion**: Water helps your body break down food and absorb nutrients.

How Much Should You Drink?

You've probably heard the advice to drink eight 8-ounce glasses of water a day. While this is a good general guideline, your actual needs may vary based on factors like:

- Your body size

- How active you are

- The climate you live in

- Your diet (some foods contain lots of water)

A good rule of thumb is to drink enough so that you rarely feel thirsty and your urine is pale yellow in color.

Hydration Strategies

1. **Start Your Day with Water**: Drink a glass of water as soon as you wake up to rehydrate after sleep.

2. **Carry a Water Bottle**: Having water easily accessible makes you more likely to drink throughout the day.

3. **Set Reminders**: If you often forget to drink, set reminders on your phone.

4. **Eat Water-Rich Foods**: Foods like cucumbers, watermelon, and soup can contribute to your fluid intake.

5. **Flavor Your Water**: If you don't like plain water, try adding slices of lemon, cucumber, or berries for natural flavor.

6. **Monitor Your Urine**: If it's dark yellow, you probably need to drink more water.

Hydration for Exercise

When you're exercising, your hydration needs increase. Here are some tips:

1. **Pre-Hydrate**: Drink about 2 cups of water 2-3 hours before exercise.

2. **During Exercise**: For workouts lasting less than an hour, water is usually sufficient. Aim to drink about 1 cup every 15-20 minutes.

3.   **For Longer Workouts**: If you're exercising intensely for more than an hour, especially in hot conditions, you might need a sports drink to replace electrolytes lost through sweat.

4.   **Post-Workout**: Drink water or a recovery beverage after your workout to replace fluids lost through sweat.

Special Considerations

- **Caffeine and Alcohol**: While these beverages do contribute to your fluid intake, they also have a mild diuretic effect. It's best not to rely on them for hydration.

- **Exercise in Heat**: When exercising in hot conditions, you'll need to drink more to compensate for increased sweating.

- **High Altitudes**: You may need to drink more water at high altitudes.

Remember, staying hydrated isn't just about drinking water during your workouts. It's about maintaining good hydration habits throughout the day, every day. Like many aspects of fitness, consistency is key when it comes to hydration. Make it a habit to sip water regularly, and your body will thank you with better performance and overall health!

5. Supplements: Necessities vs. Marketing Hype

Walk into any health food store or gym, and you'll likely see shelves full of colorful bottles promising everything from better workouts to perfect health. But do you really need supplements? Let's separate the facts from the hype and explore when supplements might be helpful and when they're just expensive urine.

What Are Supplements?

Dietary supplements are products intended to add nutrients to your diet or to lower your risk of health problems. They can include vitamins, minerals, herbs, amino acids, and enzymes. They come in various forms like pills, powders, drinks, and energy bars.

The Basics: Food First

Before we dive into specific supplements, it's important to understand a key principle: For most people, a balanced diet provides all the nutrients you need. Whole foods contain vitamins, minerals, and other beneficial compounds in forms that your body can easily use. Plus, they come packaged with fiber and other nutrients that work together in ways we don't fully understand yet.

When Might Supplements Be Necessary?

There are some situations where supplements can be beneficial:

1. **Specific Deficiencies**: If blood tests show you're low in a particular nutrient, your doctor might recommend a supplement.

2. **Pregnancy**: Pregnant women often need extra folic acid and iron.

3.   **Older Adults**: As we age, we might need more of certain nutrients, like vitamin B12 or vitamin D.

4.   **Restricted Diets**: If you're vegan or have food allergies that limit your diet, you might need certain supplements.

5.   **Certain Health Conditions**: Some health conditions can affect nutrient absorption or increase your needs for certain nutrients.

Common Supplements in the Fitness World

Let's look at some popular supplements and what science says about them:

1.   **Protein Powder**:

- What it is: Concentrated protein from sources like whey, casein, soy, or peas.

- The hype: Builds muscle, aids recovery, helps with weight loss.

- The reality: Can be convenient for meeting protein needs, especially for athletes or vegetarians. However, most people can get enough protein from food.

2.   **Creatine**:

- What it is: A compound that helps produce energy for muscle contractions.

- The hype: Increases muscle mass and strength, improves athletic performance.

- o The reality: One of the most well-researched supplements. It can be effective for high-intensity, short-duration activities like weightlifting or sprinting.

3. **Multivitamins**:

- o What they are: A combination of essential vitamins and minerals.
- o The hype: Insurance against nutrient deficiencies, better overall health.
- o The reality: While they can help fill small nutrient gaps, they're not a substitute for a healthy diet. Most people don't need them if they eat a varied diet.

4. **Fish Oil**:

- o What it is: A source of omega-3 fatty acids.
- o The hype: Improves heart health, reduces inflammation, enhances brain function.
- o The reality: Beneficial for heart health, especially if you don't eat fatty fish regularly. However, getting omega-3s from whole food sources is preferable when possible.

5. **Pre-workout Supplements**:

- o What they are: A mix of ingredients like caffeine, amino acids, and creatine.

o   The hype: Boosts energy, improves performance, enhances focus.

o   The reality: The caffeine can provide an energy boost, but many ingredients are unnecessary or under-researched. A cup of coffee can often provide similar benefits.

The Downsides of Supplements

While supplements can be beneficial in some cases, they also come with potential risks:

1. **Regulation Issues**: The supplement industry isn't as tightly regulated as pharmaceuticals. This means the quality and purity of products can vary.

2. **Interactions**: Some supplements can interact with medications or other supplements in harmful ways.

3. **Side Effects**: Even natural supplements can cause side effects, especially if taken in large doses.

4. **False Sense of Security**: Relying on supplements might lead some people to pay less attention to their overall diet.

5. **Cost**: Supplements can be expensive, and that money might be better spent on high-quality, nutritious foods.

1. **Consult a Professional**: Before starting any supplement regimen, talk to your doctor or a registered dietitian.

2. **Be Skeptical of Claims**: If it sounds too good to be true, it probably is. Be wary of products promising miraculous results.

3. **Look for Quality**: Choose supplements that have been third-party tested for quality and purity.

4. **Start with Food**: Always prioritize getting nutrients from whole foods before turning to supplements.

5. **Consider Your Needs**: Think about your specific health situation, diet, and fitness goals when considering supplements.

Remember, there's no magic pill for health and fitness. While supplements can play a role in some situations, they're just one small piece of the puzzle. A balanced diet, regular exercise, adequate sleep, and stress management are the true foundations of health and fitness.

6. Navigating Dietary Restrictions and Preferences

In today's diverse world, many people follow specific dietary patterns due to health conditions, ethical beliefs, cultural traditions, or personal preferences. Whether you're vegetarian, vegan, gluten-free, or have food allergies, it's important to know how to meet your nutritional needs while respecting your dietary choices or restrictions.

Common Dietary Restrictions and Preferences

1. **Vegetarian**: Excludes meat, often for ethical, environmental, or health reasons. There are several types:

   o Lacto-ovo vegetarians eat dairy and eggs but no meat or fish.

   o Lacto vegetarians include dairy but no eggs or meat.

   o Ovo vegetarians eat eggs but no dairy or meat.

2. **Vegan**: Excludes all animal products, including meat, dairy, eggs, and often honey.

3. **Gluten-Free**: Excludes gluten, a protein found in wheat, barley, and rye. Essential for people with celiac disease or gluten sensitivity.

4. **Dairy-Free**: Excludes milk and milk products. Necessary for people with lactose intolerance or milk allergies.

5. **Paleo**: Based on foods presumed to have been eaten by early humans, including meat, fish, vegetables, and fruit, and excluding dairy, grains, and processed foods.

6. **Keto**: Very low in carbohydrates, moderate in protein, and high in fat.

7. **Food Allergies**: May require avoiding specific foods like nuts, shellfish, or soy.

Meeting Nutritional Needs with Dietary Restrictions

Regardless of your dietary pattern, it's important to ensure you're getting all the nutrients your body needs. Here are some tips for common restrictions:

Vegetarian and Vegan Diets

- **Protein**: Include plant-based proteins like beans, lentils, tofu, tempeh, and seitan. For vegetarians, eggs and dairy are also good protein sources.

- **Iron**: Plant sources include leafy greens, beans, and fortified cereals. Eat with vitamin C-rich foods to enhance absorption.

- **Vitamin B12**: This can be challenging for vegans as it's mainly found in animal products. Look for fortified foods or consider a supplement.

- **Calcium**: For vegans, good sources include fortified plant milks, leafy greens, and calcium-set tofu.

- **Omega-3s**: Consider algae-based supplements or include walnuts, flax seeds, and chia seeds in your diet.

Gluten-Free Diet

- Focus on naturally gluten-free whole grains like rice, quinoa, and oats (ensure they're certified gluten-free).

- Be cautious of cross-contamination, especially when eating out.

- Read labels carefully, as gluten can be found in unexpected products.

- Ensure you're getting enough fiber, as many gluten-free products are lower in fiber than their wheat-based counterparts.

Dairy-Free Diet

- Calcium: Look for fortified plant milks, leafy greens, and canned fish with bones.

- Vitamin D: Consider a supplement or look for fortified foods.

- Protein: If you're not vegetarian, meat, fish, and eggs are good sources. Plant-based options include beans, nuts, and seeds.

Paleo and Keto Diets

- Ensure you're getting enough fiber from allowed vegetables and fruits.

- For keto, be mindful of getting enough micronutrients, as fruit and some vegetable intake is limited.

- Consider consulting a dietitian to ensure you're meeting all your nutritional needs.

General Tips for Navigating Dietary Restrictions

1. **Plan Ahead**: Meal planning can be especially helpful when you have dietary restrictions.

2. **Read Labels**: Ingredients you're avoiding can show up in surprising places.

3. **Communicate Clearly**: When eating out or at social gatherings, don't be afraid to ask about ingredients or preparation methods.

4. **Focus on What You Can Eat**: Instead of dwelling on foods you can't have, explore new foods and recipes that fit your diet.

5. **Be Creative with Substitutions**: There are often ways to modify recipes to fit your dietary needs.

6. **Consider Supplements**: In some cases, you might need supplements to meet all your nutritional needs. Consult with a healthcare provider or registered dietitian.

7. **Stay Balanced**: Even with restrictions, aim for a diet that includes a variety of foods from all the food groups you can eat.

Balancing Nutrition and Fitness Goals with Dietary Restrictions

When you have both specific fitness goals and dietary restrictions, it can feel challenging to meet all your needs. Here are some strategies:

1. **Consult a Professional**: A registered dietitian, especially one familiar with your specific dietary restriction and fitness goals, can be invaluable.

2. **Prioritize Protein**: Regardless of your diet, getting enough protein is crucial for fitness. If your options are limited, you might need to be more intentional about including protein sources at each meal.

3. **Don't Fear Carbs**: Unless medically necessary (like with keto for epilepsy management), remember that carbs are important for fueling workouts. Choose whole grain and high-fiber options when possible.

4. **Timing Matters**: Pay attention to when you eat, not just what you eat. This can be especially important for high-intensity training or endurance activities.

5. **Listen to Your Body**: Pay attention to how different foods make you feel during and after workouts. This can guide you in fine-tuning your diet.

6. **Be Flexible**: Sometimes, you might need to adjust your fitness routine to align with your dietary needs, or vice versa. It's all about finding a balance that works for you.

Remember, having dietary restrictions doesn't mean you can't achieve your fitness goals. It might require more planning and creativity, but with the right approach, you can fuel your body effectively while respecting your dietary choices or needs.

The key is to focus on nutrient-dense whole foods that fit within your dietary pattern, stay hydrated, and listen to your body. With some experimentation and perhaps guidance from a healthcare professional, you can find an eating pattern that supports both your dietary needs and your fitness goals.

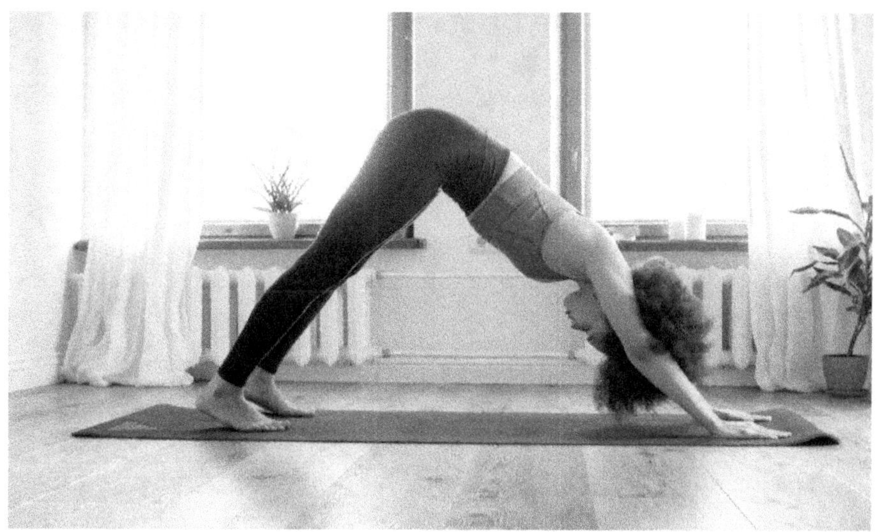

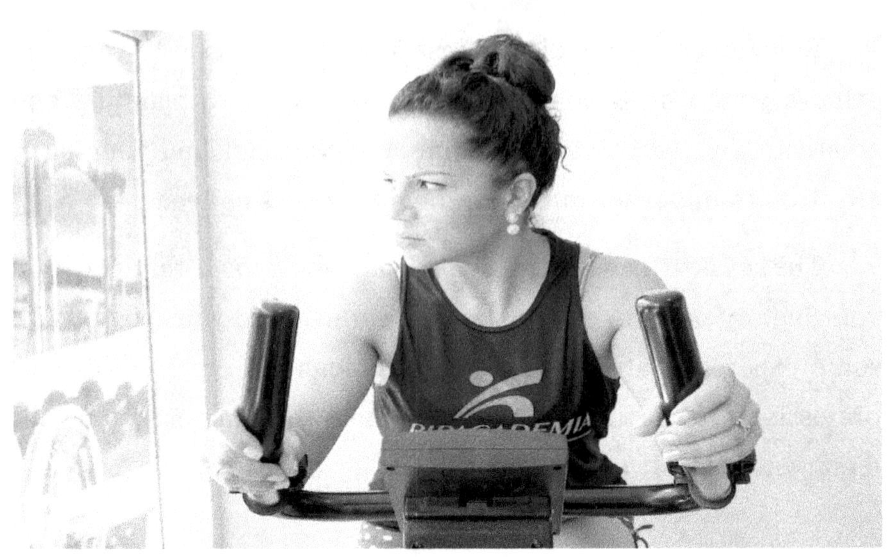

Chapter 4

Mastering Stress for Better Wellbeing

In our fast-paced world, stress has become an inevitable part of life. While some stress can be motivating and even beneficial, chronic stress can have severe consequences on our health, fitness, and overall wellbeing. This chapter will explore the stress response, its impact on our bodies, and provide practical techniques to manage stress effectively. By mastering stress management, you'll be better equipped to lead a healthier, more balanced life.

1. Understanding the Stress Response

The stress response, also known as the "fight-or-flight" response, is a natural physiological reaction that has helped humans survive for thousands of years. When we perceive a threat, our body releases stress hormones like cortisol and adrenaline, preparing us to either confront the danger or flee from it.

During this response:

- Heart rate increases

- Breathing becomes rapid

- Muscles tense up

- Blood flow is diverted to essential organs

- Digestion slows down

- Immune system function is temporarily suppressed

In prehistoric times, this response was crucial for survival against physical threats. Today, however, our stress triggers are often psychological rather than physical. Work deadlines, financial worries, and relationship issues can all activate the stress response, even when there's no immediate physical danger.

While the stress response is designed to be temporary, modern life often keeps us in a prolonged state of stress. This is where problems begin to arise.

2. The Impact of Chronic Stress on Health and Fitness

When stress becomes chronic, it can have far-reaching effects on our physical and mental health. Some of the ways chronic stress impacts our wellbeing include:

1. Cardiovascular health: Prolonged stress can lead to high blood pressure, increased risk of heart disease, and stroke.

2.   Digestive system: Stress can exacerbate conditions like acid reflux, ulcers, and irritable bowel syndrome.

3.   Immune system: Chronic stress weakens the immune system, making us more susceptible to infections and illnesses.

4.   Mental health: Stress is a significant contributor to anxiety and depression.

5.   Weight management: Stress often leads to emotional eating and can disrupt metabolism, making it harder to maintain a healthy weight.

6.   Sleep: Stress can cause insomnia and disrupt sleep patterns, leading to fatigue and decreased cognitive function.

7.   Muscle tension: Chronic stress can lead to persistent muscle tension, causing pain and discomfort.

8.   Hormonal imbalances: Prolonged stress can disrupt the balance of hormones in the body, affecting everything from mood to reproductive health.

9.   Cognitive function: Stress can impair memory, concentration, and decision-making abilities.

10.   Fitness progress: High stress levels can hinder muscle recovery, decrease motivation for exercise, and negatively impact athletic performance.

Recognizing these impacts underscores the importance of effective stress management for overall health and fitness. Let's explore some techniques to help you master your stress response.

3. Stress Management Techniques

a. Meditation and Mindfulness

Meditation and mindfulness practices have gained significant popularity in recent years, and for good reason. These techniques can help reduce stress, improve focus, and promote emotional wellbeing.

Meditation involves focusing your attention to achieve a state of calm and relaxation. There are many forms of meditation, including:

1. Mindfulness meditation: Focusing on the present moment, often by paying attention to your breath or bodily sensations.

2. Loving-kindness meditation: Cultivating feelings of compassion and goodwill towards yourself and others.

3. Transcendental meditation: Using a mantra or repeated word to achieve a state of relaxed awareness.

4. Body scan meditation: Systematically relaxing different parts of your body.

To get started with meditation:

- Find a quiet, comfortable place to sit or lie down.

- Set aside 5-10 minutes initially, gradually increasing the duration as you become more comfortable.

- Focus on your breath, a mantra, or a specific part of your body.

- When your mind wanders (which is normal), gently bring your attention back to your focus point.

Mindfulness, closely related to meditation, involves being fully present and engaged in the current moment. You can practice mindfulness throughout your day by:

- Eating mindfully, savoring each bite and paying attention to flavors and textures.

- Walking mindfully, noticing the sensation of your feet touching the ground and the environment around you.

- Listening mindfully during conversations, giving your full attention to the speaker.

Regular practice of meditation and mindfulness can help reduce stress, improve emotional regulation, and enhance overall wellbeing.

b. Breathing Exercises

Controlled breathing is a powerful tool for managing stress. It can help activate the body's relaxation response, counteracting the effects of the stress response. Here are three effective breathing techniques:

1. Deep Belly Breathing:

- o Sit or lie comfortably with one hand on your chest and the other on your belly.

- o Breathe in slowly through your nose, allowing your belly to expand while keeping your chest relatively still.

- o Exhale slowly through your mouth, feeling your belly fall.

- o Repeat for 5-10 minutes.

2. 4-7-8 Breathing:

- o Sit comfortably with your back straight.

- o Exhale completely through your mouth.

- o Close your mouth and inhale quietly through your nose for a count of 4.

- o Hold your breath for a count of 7.

- o Exhale completely through your mouth for a count of 8.

- o Repeat this cycle 3-4 times.

3. Box Breathing:

- o Sit comfortably and exhale completely.

- o Inhale through your nose for a count of 4.

- o Hold your breath for a count of 4.

- o Exhale through your mouth for a count of 4.

o   Hold your breath for a count of 4.

o   Repeat this cycle for 5-10 minutes.

Practice these techniques regularly, even when you're not feeling stressed. This will make them more effective when you need them during high-stress situations.

c. Progressive Muscle Relaxation

Progressive Muscle Relaxation (PMR) is a technique that involves systematically tensing and then relaxing different muscle groups in the body. This practice can help reduce physical tension associated with stress and promote a sense of calm. Here's how to do it:

1.   Find a quiet, comfortable place to sit or lie down.

2.   Take a few deep breaths to center yourself.

3.   Start with your feet. Tense the muscles in your feet by curling your toes and tightening your arches. Hold for 5 seconds, then release and relax for 10 seconds.

4.   Move up to your calves. Tense the muscles by pointing your toes towards your head. Hold for 5 seconds, then release and relax for 10 seconds.

5.   Continue this process, moving up through your body:

o   Thighs

o   Buttocks

o   Abdomen

o   Chest

o   Arms and hands

o   Shoulders

o   Neck

o   Face

6.   For each muscle group, tense for 5 seconds and relax for 10 seconds.

7.   After you've worked through your entire body, take a few moments to enjoy the feeling of relaxation.

Regular practice of PMR can help you become more aware of physical tension in your body and give you a tool to release it quickly.

4. The Role of Exercise in Stress Reduction

Exercise is not just crucial for physical fitness; it's also an excellent stress management tool. Regular physical activity can help reduce stress in several ways:

1.   Endorphin release: Exercise stimulates the production of endorphins, the body's natural mood elevators.

2.   Cortisol regulation: Regular exercise can help regulate cortisol levels, potentially reducing the negative effects of stress.

3.   Improved sleep: Physical activity can help improve sleep quality, which is often disrupted by stress.

4.   Increased self-confidence: Achieving fitness goals can boost self-esteem and resilience.

5.   Mindfulness opportunity: Exercise can serve as a form of moving meditation, helping you focus on the present moment.

6.   Social interaction: Group exercise classes or team sports can provide social support, which is beneficial for stress management.

To harness the stress-reducing benefits of exercise:

- Aim for at least 150 minutes of moderate-intensity aerobic activity or 75 minutes of vigorous-intensity aerobic activity per week.

- Include strength training exercises at least twice a week.

- Choose activities you enjoy to increase the likelihood of sticking with your routine.

- Consider mind-body exercises like yoga or tai chi, which combine physical activity with mindfulness.

- Use exercise as a healthy outlet for stress-related emotions like frustration or anger.

Remember, consistency is key. Even short bouts of physical activity can have mood-boosting effects, so try to incorporate movement into your daily routine.

5. Time Management and Work-Life Balance

Poor time management can be a significant source of stress. Feeling overwhelmed by tasks or constantly rushing to meet deadlines can keep your stress response activated. Here are some strategies to improve your time management and achieve better work-life balance:

1. Prioritize tasks:

    o   Use the Eisenhower Matrix to categorize tasks based on urgency and importance.

    o   Focus on high-priority tasks first.

2. Set realistic goals:

    o   Break larger projects into smaller, manageable tasks.

    o   Use the SMART criteria (Specific, Measurable, Achievable, Relevant, Time-bound) when setting goals.

3. Use time-blocking:

    o   Allocate specific time slots for different tasks or types of work.

    o   Include breaks in your schedule to avoid burnout.

4. Minimize distractions:

    o   Identify your biggest time-wasters (e.g., social media, unnecessary meetings).

    o   Use tools like website blockers or "Do Not Disturb" modes on your devices.

5.   Learn to say "no":

    o   Be selective about which commitments you take on.

    o   Politely decline requests that don't align with your priorities or values.

6.   Delegate when possible:

    o   At work, delegate tasks to team members when appropriate.

    o   At home, share responsibilities with family members.

7.   Create boundaries between work and personal life:

    o   Establish a dedicated workspace if working from home.

    o   Set clear "office hours" and stick to them.

    o   Avoid checking work emails during personal time.

8.   Practice self-care:

    o   Schedule time for activities you enjoy.

    o   Prioritize sleep, healthy eating, and exercise.

9.   Use productivity techniques:

> o   Try methods like the Pomodoro Technique (25 minutes of focused work followed by a 5-minute break).
>
> o   Experiment with different productivity apps or tools to find what works best for you.

10.   Regularly reassess and adjust:

> o   Review your time management strategies periodically.
>
> o   Be willing to adjust your approach based on what's working and what's not.

Remember, the goal of time management isn't to fill every moment with productivity. It's about creating a balanced life where you have time for work, relationships, personal growth, and relaxation.

6. Building Resilience Through Positive Psychology

Resilience is the ability to bounce back from stress, adversity, and challenges. It's not about avoiding stress entirely (which is impossible), but about developing the mental and emotional tools to cope effectively with stress. Positive psychology, which focuses on cultivating strengths and positive emotions, offers several strategies for building resilience:

1.   Cultivate optimism:

- o   Practice looking for the silver lining in difficult situations.
- o   Challenge negative self-talk with more balanced, realistic thoughts.

2.   Develop a growth mindset:

- o   View challenges as opportunities for learning and growth.
- o   Embrace the phrase "not yet" when facing difficulties.

3.   Practice gratitude:

- o   Keep a gratitude journal, writing down three things you're thankful for each day.
- o   Express appreciation to others regularly.

4.   Build strong relationships:

- o   Invest time in nurturing supportive relationships.
- o   Reach out to others during times of stress.

5.   Find meaning and purpose:

- o   Clarify your personal values and align your actions with them.
- o   Engage in activities that give you a sense of purpose.

6. Develop emotional intelligence:

- o Practice identifying and naming your emotions.
- o Learn healthy ways to express and manage your feelings.

7. Practice self-compassion:

- o Treat yourself with the same kindness you'd offer a good friend.
- o Avoid harsh self-criticism, especially during stressful times.

8. Engage in acts of kindness:

- o Look for opportunities to help others.
- o Volunteer for causes you care about.

9. Cultivate mindfulness:

- o Practice being present in the moment without judgment.
- o Incorporate mindfulness into daily activities.

10. Focus on your strengths:

- o Identify your personal strengths and find ways to use them more often.
- o Approach challenges by leveraging your strengths.

11. Set and pursue goals:

o Having clear, meaningful goals can provide direction and motivation.

o Celebrate small victories along the way to larger goals.

12.   Practice problem-solving:

o Approach stressors as problems to be solved rather than insurmountable obstacles.

o Break down complex issues into manageable steps.

Building resilience is an ongoing process. It involves developing a set of skills and mindsets that allow you to navigate life's challenges more effectively. By incorporating these positive psychology strategies into your life, you can enhance your ability to manage stress and maintain wellbeing even in difficult times.

In conclusion, mastering stress is essential for maintaining optimal health, fitness, and overall wellbeing. By understanding the stress response, recognizing the impact of chronic stress, and implementing effective stress management techniques, you can significantly improve your quality of life. Remember that managing stress is a skill that improves with practice. Be patient with yourself as you explore different strategies and find what works best for you. With time and consistent effort, you'll develop greater resilience and the ability to thrive even in challenging circumstances.

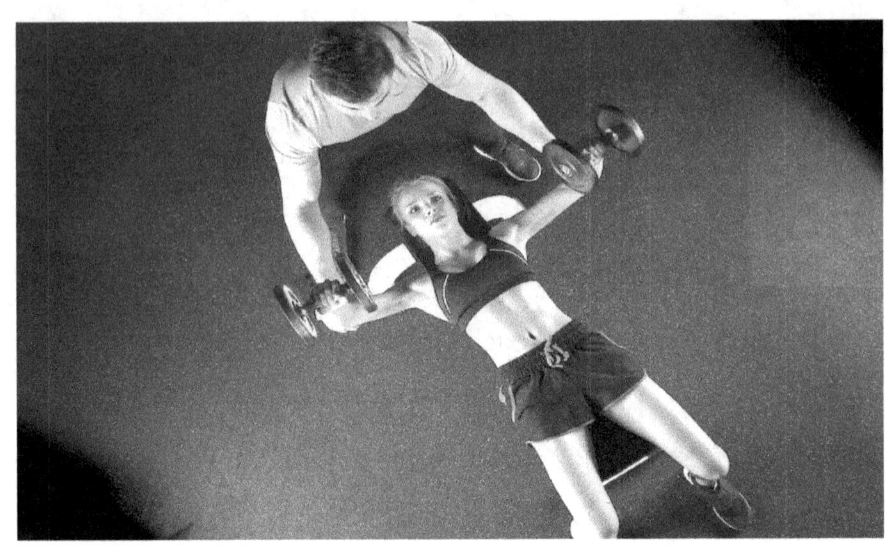

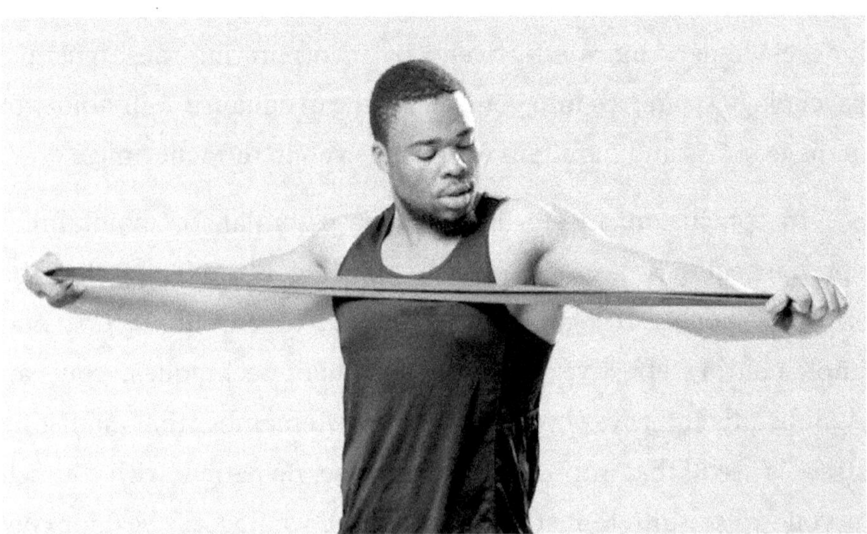

Chapter 5

Understanding and Implementing Various Exercise Types

Exercise is a cornerstone of a healthy lifestyle, offering numerous benefits for both physical and mental well-being. However, with the vast array of exercise types available, it can be overwhelming to know where to start or how to create a well-rounded fitness routine. This chapter will explore various exercise types, their benefits, and how to implement them effectively in your fitness journey.

1. Cardiovascular Exercise

Cardiovascular exercise, often referred to as cardio or aerobic exercise, is any activity that increases your heart rate and breathing for an extended period. This type of exercise is crucial for heart health, endurance, and overall fitness.

a. Benefits and Types

Benefits of cardiovascular exercise include:

1.   Improved heart health

2.   Increased lung capacity

3.   Better circulation

4.   Weight management

5.   Reduced risk of chronic diseases

6.   Enhanced mood and mental health

7.   Increased energy levels

8.   Better sleep quality

Types of cardiovascular exercise:

1.   Running/Jogging

2.   Brisk walking

3.   Cycling

4.   Swimming

5.   Dancing

6.   Rowing

7.   Jumping rope

8.   Stair climbing

9.   Elliptical training

10.   Cross-country skiing

Each type of cardio offers unique benefits and engages different muscle groups. For example, swimming is a low-impact full-body workout, while running provides a high-impact lower body focus.

b. How to Create an Effective Cardio Routine

To create an effective cardiovascular routine:

1. Assess your current fitness level: Begin with activities that match your ability and gradually increase intensity.

2. Set clear goals: Determine what you want to achieve (e.g., weight loss, improved endurance, or better overall health).

3. Choose activities you enjoy: You're more likely to stick with exercises you find fun or engaging.

4. Vary your routine: Incorporate different types of cardio to prevent boredom and work different muscle groups.

5. Follow the FITT principle:

   - Frequency: Aim for at least 150 minutes of moderate-intensity or 75 minutes of vigorous-intensity cardio per week.

   - Intensity: Work at a level that elevates your heart rate to 50-85% of your maximum heart rate.

   - Time: Start with shorter sessions (10-15 minutes) and gradually increase duration.

   - Type: Choose activities that suit your preferences and fitness goals.

6. Incorporate interval training: Alternate between high and low-intensity periods to boost cardiovascular fitness and calorie burn.

7. Warm up and cool down: Always include 5-10 minutes of light activity before and after your main workout.

8. Monitor your progress: Keep track of your workouts and adjust as needed.

9. Listen to your body: Rest when needed and avoid overtraining.

Remember, consistency is key. It's better to do moderate exercise regularly than to push too hard infrequently and risk injury or burnout.

2. Strength Training

Strength training, also known as resistance training, involves working against a force to build muscle strength, size, and endurance. It's a crucial component of any well-rounded fitness program.

a. Benefits of Resistance Training

1. Increased muscle mass and strength

2. Improved bone density

3. Enhanced metabolic rate

4. Better body composition (more lean muscle, less fat)

5. Improved functional fitness for daily activities

6.   Reduced risk of injury

7.   Enhanced athletic performance

8.   Better glucose metabolism and insulin sensitivity

9.   Improved posture and balance

10.   Increased confidence and body image

b. Basic Principles of Weightlifting

To get the most out of your strength training, follow these principles:

1.   Progressive overload: Gradually increase the weight, frequency, or number of repetitions to continually challenge your muscles.

2.   Specificity: Target exercises to your specific goals (e.g., focus on compound movements for overall strength, isolation exercises for specific muscle groups).

3.   Rest and recovery: Allow adequate time between workouts for muscles to repair and grow stronger.

4.   Proper form: Maintain correct technique to maximize benefits and minimize injury risk.

5.   Balanced routine: Work all major muscle groups for overall strength and symmetry.

6.   Variation: Regularly change exercises, rep ranges, and training methods to prevent plateaus.

7.   Consistency: Regular workouts are key to seeing progress.

8. Proper nutrition: Support your training with adequate protein, carbohydrates, and overall calorie intake.

When starting a weightlifting routine:

1. Begin with a full-body workout 2-3 times per week.

2. Focus on compound exercises that work multiple muscle groups:

    o Squats

    o Deadlifts

    o Bench presses

    o Rows

    o Overhead presses

3. Start with light weights to perfect your form.

4. Aim for 2-3 sets of 8-12 repetitions for each exercise.

5. Gradually increase weight as you become stronger.

6. Always use proper safety equipment and techniques, such as weight belts for heavy lifts and spotters when necessary.

c. Bodyweight Exercises for Beginners

Bodyweight exercises are an excellent way to start strength training, requiring no equipment and easily adaptable to different fitness levels. Here are some effective bodyweight exercises for beginners:

1. Push-ups: Work chest, shoulders, and triceps.

2. Squats: Target legs and core.

3.   Lunges: Focus on legs and improve balance.

4.   Plank: Strengthens core and improves posture.

5.   Burpees: Full-body exercise that also provides cardiovascular benefits.

6.   Mountain climbers: Work core and provide cardio.

7.   Dips: Target triceps and chest.

8.   Glute bridges: Strengthen glutes and lower back.

9.   Wall sits: Isometric exercise for legs.

10.   Superman: Targets lower back and core.

Start with 2-3 sets of 8-12 repetitions for each exercise, focusing on proper form. As you get stronger, increase the number of repetitions or try more challenging variations of each exercise.

3. Flexibility and Mobility Work

Flexibility and mobility are often overlooked components of fitness, but they play a crucial role in overall health and performance.

a. The Importance of Stretching

Stretching offers numerous benefits:

1.   Improved flexibility and range of motion

2.   Reduced risk of injury

3.   Better posture

4.   Decreased muscle tension and soreness

5.   Enhanced athletic performance

6.   Improved blood flow and circulation

7.   Stress relief and relaxation

b. Types of Stretching

1.   Static Stretching:

- Involves holding a stretch for 15-60 seconds.
- Best performed after workouts or as a separate flexibility session.
- Examples: Hamstring stretch, quad stretch, shoulder stretch.

2.   Dynamic Stretching:

- Involves moving parts of your body and gradually increasing reach, speed of movement, or both.
- Ideal for pre-workout warm-ups.
- Examples: Leg swings, arm circles, walking lunges.

3.   PNF (Proprioceptive Neuromuscular Facilitation) Stretching:

- Involves alternating contraction and relaxation of muscle groups.

o   Often requires a partner or specialized equipment.

o   Can lead to rapid flexibility gains but should be performed carefully to avoid injury.

4.   Ballistic Stretching:

o   Involves bouncing or jerking movements to push a body part beyond its normal range of motion.

o   Generally not recommended due to increased injury risk.

c. Yoga and Pilates for Flexibility

Yoga and Pilates are excellent practices for improving flexibility, balance, and core strength.

Yoga:

- Combines physical postures, breathing techniques, and meditation.

- Offers various styles from gentle (e.g., Hatha) to more vigorous (e.g., Vinyasa, Ashtanga).

- Benefits include improved flexibility, strength, balance, and stress reduction.

Pilates:

- Focuses on core strength, posture, and controlled movements.

- Can be done on a mat or with specialized equipment like the Reformer.

- Enhances flexibility, core strength, and body awareness.

Both practices can be adapted for all fitness levels and are excellent complements to other forms of exercise.

4. High-Intensity Interval Training (HIIT)

High-Intensity Interval Training (HIIT) has gained popularity due to its efficiency and effectiveness in improving both cardiovascular fitness and muscle strength.

What is HIIT?

- Short bursts of high-intensity exercise alternated with periods of lower-intensity exercise or rest.

- Can be applied to various types of exercise (e.g., running, cycling, bodyweight exercises).

- Typically lasts 10-30 minutes.

Benefits of HIIT:

1. Efficient calorie burn

2. Improved cardiovascular fitness

3. Enhanced metabolic rate

4. Increased fat loss

5.   Muscle preservation during weight loss

6.   No equipment necessary (though it can be used)

7.   Challenging and varied workouts

Sample HIIT Workout:

1.   Warm-up: 5 minutes of light jogging or marching in place

2.   30 seconds of high-intensity exercise (e.g., burpees)

3.   30 seconds of low-intensity exercise (e.g., walking in place)

4.   Repeat steps 2-3 for a total of 15-20 minutes

5.   Cool-down: 5 minutes of light stretching

When incorporating HIIT:

- Start with once or twice a week, allowing for recovery between sessions.

- Gradually increase intensity and frequency as your fitness improves.

- Always warm up properly and maintain good form to prevent injury.

- Listen to your body and adjust intensity as needed.

5. Sports and Recreational Activities as Fitness Tools

Engaging in sports and recreational activities can be an enjoyable way to improve fitness while developing skills and social connections.

Benefits of sports and recreational activities:

1. Improved cardiovascular fitness

2. Enhanced strength and flexibility

3. Better coordination and balance

4. Stress relief and mental health benefits

5. Social interaction and teamwork skills

6. Goal-setting and achievement

7. Fun and enjoyment, leading to better adherence

Popular sports and activities for fitness:

1. Tennis: Improves cardiovascular fitness, agility, and hand-eye coordination.

2. Basketball: Enhances endurance, speed, and teamwork skills.

3. Soccer: Boosts cardiovascular fitness, leg strength, and coordination.

4. Swimming: Provides a full-body, low-impact workout.

5. Rock climbing: Builds upper body and core strength, as well as problem-solving skills.

6. Martial arts: Improves flexibility, strength, and mental focus.

7.   Dancing: Enhances coordination, balance, and cardiovascular fitness.

8.   Hiking: Builds leg strength and endurance while connecting with nature.

When using sports for fitness:

- Choose activities you enjoy to ensure long-term adherence.

- Gradually increase intensity and duration to avoid injury.

- Incorporate proper warm-up and cool-down routines.

- Consider cross-training with other activities to ensure balanced fitness.

- Don't forget to include rest days for recovery.

6. Creating a Balanced Exercise Program

A well-rounded fitness program should incorporate various types of exercise to ensure overall health and fitness. Here's how to create a balanced exercise program:

1.   Assess your current fitness level and goals:

    o   Consider your strengths, weaknesses, and any health concerns.

- Set SMART goals (Specific, Measurable, Achievable, Relevant, Time-bound).

2. Include all components of fitness:

   - Cardiovascular endurance

   - Muscular strength and endurance

   - Flexibility and mobility

   - Balance and coordination

3. Follow general exercise guidelines:

   - Aim for at least 150 minutes of moderate-intensity or 75 minutes of vigorous-intensity aerobic activity per week.

   - Perform strength training exercises for all major muscle groups at least twice a week.

   - Include flexibility work daily, with more focused sessions 2-3 times per week.

4. Structure your week:

   - Monday: Strength training (full body) + short HIIT session

   - Tuesday: Moderate-intensity cardio (e.g., jogging, cycling)

   - Wednesday: Yoga or Pilates

   - Thursday: Strength training (full body) + short HIIT session

- o   Friday: Sports or recreational activity

- o   Saturday: Longer cardio session (e.g., hike, swim)

- o   Sunday: Active recovery (light walk, stretching)

5. Apply progressive overload:

- o   Gradually increase the challenge of your workouts over time.

- o   This can involve increasing weight, reps, duration, or intensity.

6. Include variety:

- o   Change up your routine every 4-6 weeks to prevent plateaus and boredom.

- o   Try new activities or exercise classes to keep things interesting.

7. Allow for proper rest and recovery:

- o   Include at least one full rest day per week.

- o   Ensure adequate sleep (7-9 hours per night for most adults).

- o   Consider active recovery activities like light walking or yoga on rest days.

8. Listen to your body:

- o   Pay attention to signs of overtraining or injury.

o   Adjust your program as needed based on how you feel.

9.   Nutrition and hydration:

o   Support your exercise program with a balanced diet.

o   Stay properly hydrated before, during, and after workouts.

10.   Track your progress:

o   Keep a workout log to monitor improvements.

o   Regularly reassess your goals and adjust your program accordingly.

11.   Seek professional guidance:

o   Consider working with a certified personal trainer or coach, especially when starting out or trying new types of exercise.

o   Consult with a healthcare provider before starting a new exercise program, particularly if you have any health concerns or conditions.

Remember, the best exercise program is one that you enjoy and can stick to consistently. Don't be afraid to adjust your routine based on your preferences, schedule, and progress. The key is to find a balance that challenges you while still being sustainable in the long term.

As you become more comfortable with different types of exercise, you can further customize your program to align with your specific goals, whether that's building muscle, improving endurance, losing weight, or enhancing overall health and wellness.

By incorporating a variety of exercise types into your routine, you'll not only see improvements in your physical fitness but also enjoy the mental and emotional benefits that come with a well-rounded approach to exercise. Stay consistent, be patient with your progress, and most importantly, have fun on your fitness journey!

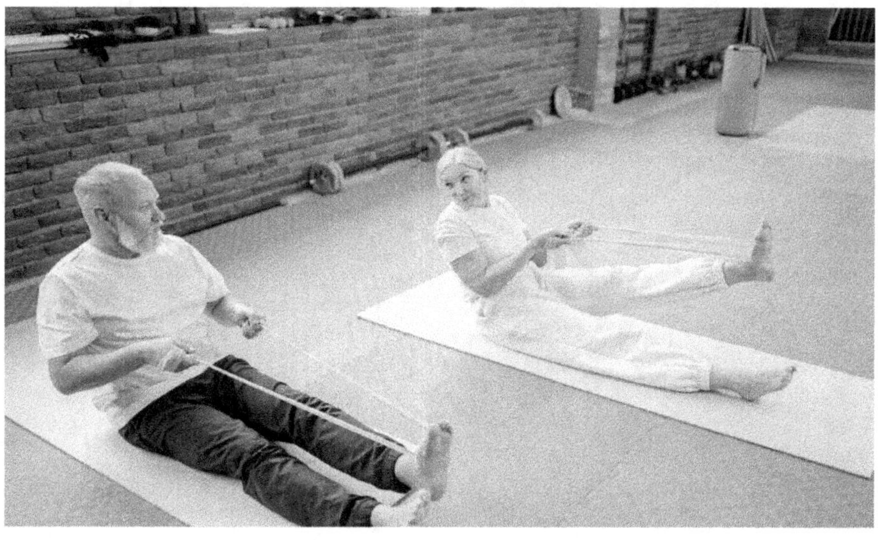

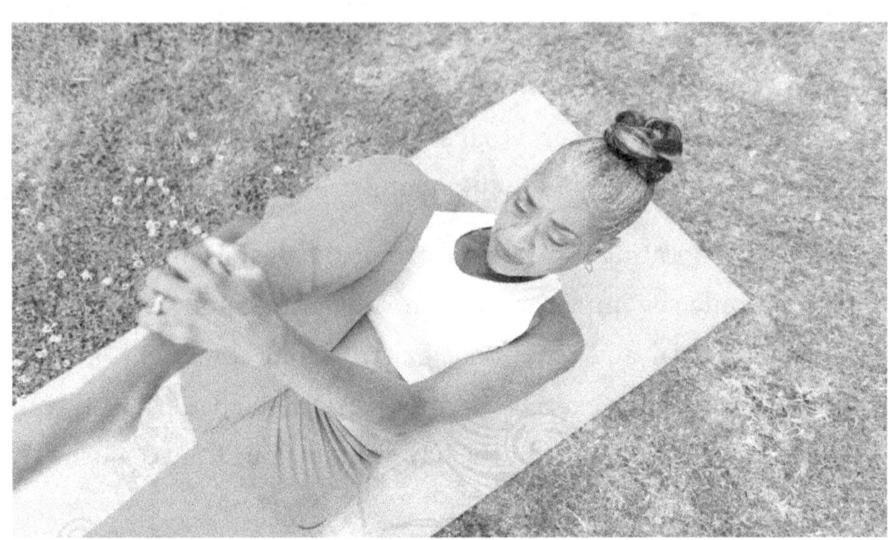

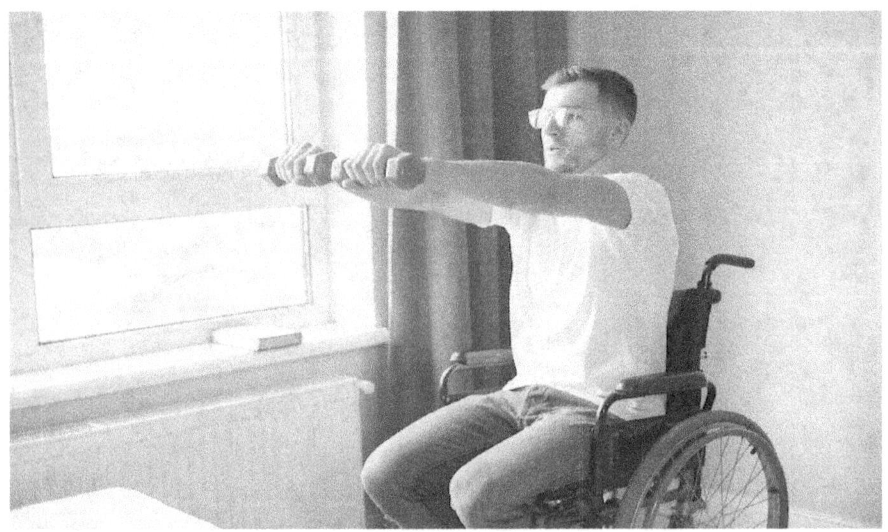

Chapter 6

Fitness Strategies for Seniors and Those with Limited Mobility

As we age or face mobility challenges, maintaining an active lifestyle becomes increasingly important. Regular exercise can help manage health conditions, improve quality of life, and promote independence. This chapter explores fitness strategies tailored for seniors and individuals with limited mobility, offering safe and effective ways to stay active and healthy.

1. Understanding Age-Related Changes in the Body

As we grow older, our bodies undergo various changes that can affect our ability to exercise and stay fit. Understanding these changes is crucial for developing appropriate fitness strategies:

1. Muscle Mass and Strength: Starting around age 30, we begin to lose muscle mass and strength, a process called

sarcopenia. This loss accelerates after age 60, leading to decreased strength and mobility.

2. Bone Density: Bones become less dense and more fragile with age, increasing the risk of osteoporosis and fractures.

3. Joint Flexibility: Joints may become stiffer and less flexible, reducing range of motion and increasing the risk of injury.

4. Balance and Coordination: The body's balance systems can deteriorate, leading to an increased risk of falls.

5. Cardiovascular System: The heart becomes less efficient at pumping blood, and blood vessels may lose some elasticity, affecting endurance and recovery time.

6. Metabolism: Metabolic rate tends to slow down, which can lead to weight gain if calorie intake isn't adjusted.

7. Immune Function: The immune system may become less effective, increasing susceptibility to illness and prolonging recovery times.

8. Sensory Changes: Vision and hearing may decline, affecting balance and spatial awareness.

9. Nervous System: Reflexes may slow, and nerve conduction can decrease, affecting reaction time and coordination.

10. Hydration: The body's ability to conserve water decreases, increasing the risk of dehydration.

These changes don't mean that staying fit is impossible; rather, they underscore the importance of tailoring exercise programs to address these specific challenges and maintain overall health and functionality.

2. Benefits of Exercise for Older Adults

Regular physical activity offers numerous benefits for seniors and those with limited mobility:

1. Improved Cardiovascular Health: Exercise strengthens the heart and improves circulation, reducing the risk of heart disease and stroke.

2. Better Management of Chronic Conditions: Physical activity can help manage conditions like diabetes, arthritis, and high blood pressure.

3. Enhanced Bone and Muscle Strength: Weight-bearing exercises and strength training help maintain bone density and muscle mass, reducing the risk of osteoporosis and falls.

4. Improved Balance and Coordination: Regular exercise enhances proprioception and balance, decreasing the likelihood of falls and injuries.

5. Weight Management: Physical activity helps maintain a healthy weight by burning calories and boosting metabolism.

6. Cognitive Function: Exercise has been shown to improve memory, reduce the risk of cognitive decline, and potentially delay the onset of dementia.

7.   Better Sleep: Regular physical activity can improve sleep quality and duration.

8.   Mood Enhancement: Exercise releases endorphins, which can help alleviate symptoms of depression and anxiety.

9.   Increased Energy Levels: Regular activity can boost overall energy and reduce fatigue.

10.   Greater Independence: By improving strength, flexibility, and balance, exercise helps seniors maintain their ability to perform daily activities independently.

11.   Social Interaction: Group exercise classes or activities provide opportunities for social engagement, which is crucial for mental health.

12.   Improved Digestive Function: Physical activity can help regulate bowel movements and reduce constipation, a common issue among older adults.

These benefits highlight why it's never too late to start exercising, even for those who have been inactive or have mobility limitations.

3. Safe Exercise Options for Seniors

When designing an exercise program for seniors or those with limited mobility, safety should be the top priority. Here are some safe and effective exercise options:

a. Low-Impact Cardiovascular Exercises

1. Walking: A simple yet effective exercise that can be done indoors or outdoors. Use a treadmill, walk in a mall, or enjoy nature trails.

2. Swimming or Water Aerobics: The buoyancy of water reduces stress on joints while providing resistance for a full-body workout.

3. Stationary Cycling: Whether using a traditional stationary bike or a recumbent bike for better back support, cycling is easy on the joints while improving cardiovascular fitness.

4. Elliptical Machines: These provide a low-impact cardiovascular workout that's gentler on the joints than running.

5. Chair Exercises: For those with very limited mobility, exercises performed while seated can still provide cardiovascular benefits.

6. Tai Chi: This gentle, flowing exercise improves balance, flexibility, and mental well-being.

Remember to start slowly and gradually increase duration and intensity. Aim for at least 150 minutes of moderate-intensity aerobic activity per week, or as much as your abilities and health allow.

b. Strength Training for Bone Health

Strength training is crucial for maintaining muscle mass and bone density. Here are some safe options:

1. Bodyweight Exercises: Squats, wall push-ups, and leg raises can be effective and require no equipment.

2. Resistance Bands: These versatile tools provide adjustable resistance for a variety of exercises.

3. Light Dumbbells or Wrist Weights: Start with light weights and focus on proper form.

4. Weight Machines: If available, weight machines can provide a controlled environment for strength training.

5. Yoga: Many yoga poses build strength while improving flexibility and balance.

Key exercises to include:

- Leg Press or Squats: Strengthens legs and core.

- Chest Press: Improves upper body strength.

- Row: Works the back muscles and improves posture.

- Shoulder Press: Enhances upper body strength and shoulder mobility.

- Hip Abduction/Adduction: Strengthens hip muscles for better stability.

Aim for 2-3 strength training sessions per week, allowing for rest days in between.

c. Balance Exercises for Fall Prevention

Improving balance is crucial for preventing falls. Incorporate these exercises:

1.   Single Leg Stand: Hold onto a chair and stand on one leg for up to 30 seconds.

2.   Heel-to-Toe Walk: Walk in a straight line, placing the heel of one foot directly in front of the toes of the other foot.

3.   Sit-to-Stand: Practice standing up from a seated position without using your hands.

4.   Clock Reach: Imagine a clock on the floor and reach to different "hours" with your foot.

5.   Balancing Wand: Balance a cane or rolled-up newspaper on your palm while walking.

6.   Tai Chi: Many Tai Chi movements inherently improve balance.

Perform balance exercises 2-3 times a week, or even daily if possible. Always have a stable support nearby when practicing these exercises.

4. Adaptations for Common Health Conditions

Many seniors and individuals with limited mobility have underlying health conditions that require special considerations. Here are some adaptations for common conditions:

1.   Arthritis:

   o   Focus on low-impact activities like swimming or cycling.

- o   Use heat therapy before exercise to loosen joints.

- o   Incorporate range-of-motion exercises to maintain flexibility.

2.   Osteoporosis:

- o   Emphasize weight-bearing exercises to strengthen bones.

- o   Avoid high-impact activities or exercises that involve bending forward from the waist.

- o   Include balance training to prevent falls.

3.   Heart Disease:

- o   Monitor intensity using the Rating of Perceived Exertion (RPE) scale.

- o   Start with shorter sessions and gradually increase duration.

- o   Include cool-down periods to prevent sudden drops in blood pressure.

4.   Diabetes:

- o   Monitor blood sugar before, during, and after exercise.

- o   Wear proper footwear to prevent foot injuries.

- o   Stay well-hydrated during workouts.

5.   Parkinson's Disease:

o   Focus on big, exaggerated movements to combat the tendency for smaller movements.

o   Include exercises that challenge balance and coordination.

o   Try rhythmic activities like dance to improve mobility.

6.   Stroke:

o   Work with a physical therapist to design appropriate exercises.

o   Focus on exercises that promote symmetry and combat one-sided weakness.

o   Include activities that challenge cognitive function along with physical movement.

7.   Chronic Obstructive Pulmonary Disease (COPD):

o   Incorporate breathing exercises into the routine.

o   Use interval training to allow for rest periods.

o   Focus on upper body exercises to improve respiratory muscle strength.

Always consult with a healthcare provider before starting a new exercise program, especially when dealing with chronic health conditions.

5. Staying Motivated and Consistent

Maintaining motivation can be challenging, but it's crucial for reaping the long-term benefits of exercise. Here are strategies to stay motivated:

1. Set Realistic Goals: Start with small, achievable goals and gradually increase the challenge.

2. Track Progress: Keep a log of your activities and celebrate small victories.

3. Find Enjoyable Activities: Choose exercises you genuinely enjoy to make fitness more fun.

4. Create a Routine: Establish a regular exercise schedule to build a habit.

5. Use Technology: Fitness trackers or smartphone apps can provide motivation and track progress.

6. Join Group Classes: Exercising with others can make workouts more enjoyable and provide accountability.

7. Reward Yourself: Set up a reward system for reaching your fitness goals.

8. Educate Yourself: Learn about the benefits of exercise to reinforce your motivation.

9. Adapt to Setbacks: If you miss a workout, don't be discouraged. Just get back on track with your next scheduled session.

10.   Visualize Success: Imagine how you'll feel and what you'll be able to do as you become more fit.

Remember, consistency is key. It's better to do a little bit regularly than to overdo it occasionally and risk burnout or injury.

6. The Importance of Social Support in Senior Fitness

Social support plays a crucial role in maintaining a consistent fitness routine, especially for seniors. Here's why it's important and how to cultivate it:

1.   Motivation and Accountability:

- Exercise partners or groups can provide encouragement and help you stick to your routine.
- Knowing others are expecting you can be a powerful motivator to show up for workouts.

2.   Safety:

- Having a workout buddy means there's someone to assist if needed and to watch out for potential hazards.
- Group classes often have instructors who can ensure exercises are performed safely.

3.   Enjoyment:

- Social interaction during exercise can make the experience more enjoyable.
- Time often passes more quickly when you're exercising with others.

4. Cognitive Benefits:

- Social interaction combined with physical activity provides dual benefits for brain health.
- Discussing workout plans or progress engages cognitive functions.

5. Emotional Support:

- Sharing fitness journeys can create bonds and provide emotional support.
- Group settings can combat feelings of isolation or loneliness common among seniors.

6. Skill Sharing:

- In group settings, participants can learn from each other's experiences and techniques.
- Diverse groups may introduce you to new types of exercises or approaches to fitness.

Ways to incorporate social support into your fitness routine:

1. Join Senior-Focused Fitness Classes: Many gyms and community centers offer classes specifically designed for older adults.

2.   Find a Walking Group: Walking groups are a great way to combine exercise with social interaction.

3.   Participate in Community Sports: Activities like golf, bowling, or pickleball can provide both exercise and social engagement.

4.   Use Technology: For those unable to leave home easily, online fitness communities or virtual classes can provide social connection.

5.   Involve Family Members: Exercise with children or grandchildren for intergenerational bonding.

6.   Volunteer: Many volunteer activities, like community gardening or leading tours at local attractions, combine physical activity with social interaction.

7.   Join a Club: Consider clubs focused on active hobbies like hiking, dancing, or birdwatching.

Remember, the goal is to create a supportive environment that encourages regular physical activity while also nurturing social connections. This combination can significantly enhance both physical and mental well-being for seniors and those with limited mobility.

In conclusion, staying active as we age or when facing mobility challenges is not just possible, but essential for maintaining health, independence, and quality of life. By understanding the changes our bodies undergo, recognizing the immense benefits of exercise, and implementing safe and enjoyable fitness strategies, seniors and individuals with limited mobility can lead active, healthy lives.

Remember to consult with healthcare providers before starting any new exercise program, especially if you have underlying health conditions. With the right approach and support, fitness can be a rewarding and enriching part of life at any age or ability level.

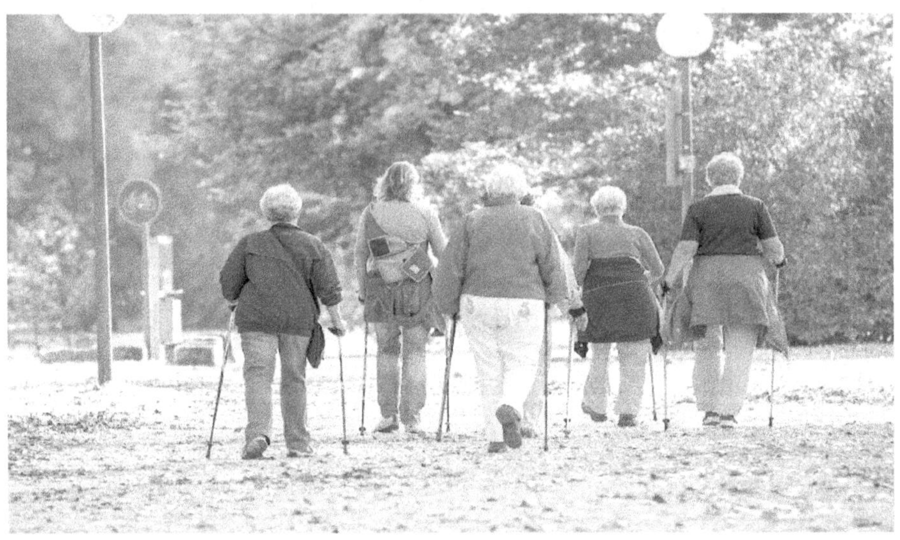

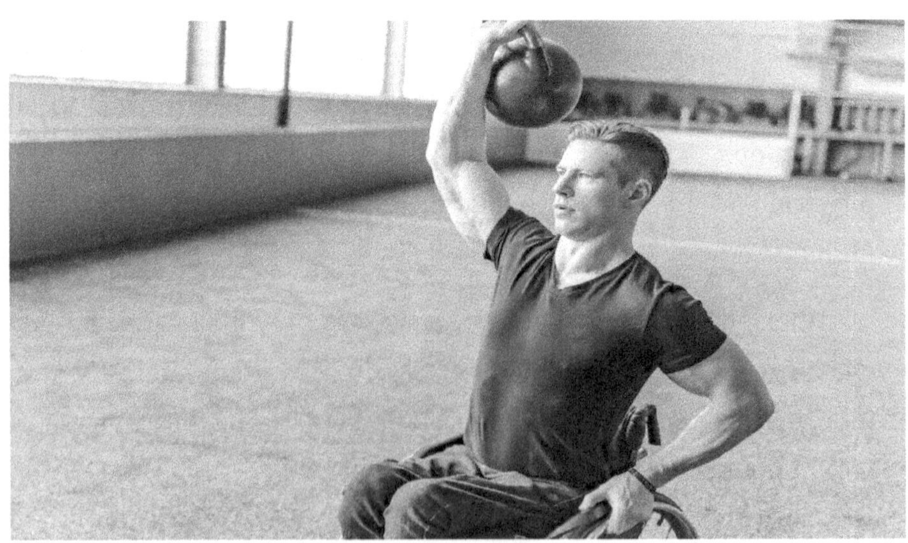

Chapter 7

The Psychology of Fitness

While physical exercise is crucial for maintaining health and fitness, the mental aspects of adopting and maintaining a fitness routine are equally important. This chapter explores the psychological factors that influence our fitness journey, providing insights and strategies to help you build a sustainable and enjoyable fitness lifestyle.

1. Understanding Motivation and Adherence

Motivation is the driving force behind our fitness goals, while adherence refers to our ability to stick to a fitness plan over time. Understanding these concepts is crucial for long-term success in any fitness endeavor.

Types of Motivation

1. Intrinsic Motivation: This comes from within and is based on personal enjoyment or satisfaction. For example, exercising because you find it fun or challenging.

2. Extrinsic Motivation: This comes from external factors, such as rewards or avoiding punishment. For example, exercising to win a competition or to avoid health problems.

While both types of motivation can be effective, research suggests that intrinsic motivation is more likely to lead to long-term adherence to a fitness routine.

Factors Affecting Motivation and Adherence

1. Goal Setting: Clear, specific, and achievable goals can significantly boost motivation.

2. Perceived Benefits: Understanding the personal benefits of exercise can increase motivation.

3. Self-Efficacy: Belief in one's ability to succeed in specific situations affects motivation and adherence.

4. Social Support: Encouragement from friends, family, or a fitness community can enhance motivation.

5. Enjoyment: Finding activities you genuinely enjoy increases the likelihood of adherence.

6. Convenience: Easy access to exercise facilities or equipment can improve adherence.

7. Past Experiences: Positive past experiences with exercise can boost motivation, while negative experiences may hinder it.

Strategies to Enhance Motivation and Adherence

1. Set SMART Goals: Specific, Measurable, Achievable, Relevant, and Time-bound goals provide clear direction.

2.   Find Your "Why": Identify deep, personal reasons for wanting to improve your fitness.

3.   Start Small: Begin with manageable changes to build confidence and momentum.

4.   Track Progress: Use a fitness journal or app to monitor improvements and celebrate small wins.

5.   Vary Your Routine: Introduce new exercises or activities to prevent boredom.

6.   Schedule Workouts: Treat exercise as an important appointment in your calendar.

7.   Reward Yourself: Establish a reward system for reaching fitness milestones.

Remember, motivation can fluctuate. The key is to develop strategies that help you stay consistent even when motivation is low.

2. Overcoming Mental Barriers to Exercise

Mental barriers can significantly impede our fitness journey. Recognizing and addressing these barriers is crucial for long-term success.

Common Mental Barriers:

1.   Lack of Time: Often cited as the primary reason for not exercising.

2. Fear of Failure: Worry about not meeting personal or others' expectations.

3. Low Self-Efficacy: Doubt in one's ability to perform exercises correctly or achieve fitness goals.

4. Body Image Issues: Feeling self-conscious about one's appearance in workout settings.

5. All-or-Nothing Thinking: Believing that if you can't do a "perfect" workout, it's not worth doing at all.

6. Overwhelm: Feeling intimidated by the perceived complexity of starting a fitness routine.

7. Negative Past Experiences: Previous unpleasant experiences with exercise creating aversion.

8. Comparison: Unfavorable comparisons to others leading to discouragement.

Strategies to Overcome Mental Barriers:

1. Reframe "Lack of Time":

   o Break exercise into smaller, manageable chunks throughout the day.

   o Prioritize exercise by scheduling it like any other important appointment.

   o Combine exercise with other activities (e.g., walking meetings, active commuting).

2. Address Fear of Failure:

- Set realistic, achievable goals to build confidence.

    - Focus on the process rather than just the outcome.

    - Redefine "failure" as a learning opportunity rather than a personal shortcoming.

3. Boost Self-Efficacy:

    - Start with exercises you feel confident performing.

    - Gradually increase difficulty as you build skills and confidence.

    - Seek guidance from fitness professionals to ensure proper form.

4. Tackle Body Image Issues:

    - Focus on how exercise makes you feel rather than how you look.

    - Choose workout environments where you feel comfortable.

    - Practice self-compassion and positive self-talk.

5. Combat All-or-Nothing Thinking:

    - Embrace the idea that any exercise is better than no exercise.

- o   Celebrate small victories and incremental progress.

- o   Create flexible workout plans that accommodate life's unpredictability.

6.   Overcome Overwhelm:

- o   Start with simple, enjoyable activities.

- o   Gradually introduce new exercises or increase intensity over time.

- o   Break down fitness goals into smaller, manageable steps.

7.   Address Negative Past Experiences:

- o   Try different types of exercise to find activities you enjoy.

- o   Focus on the positive aspects of exercise, such as increased energy or stress relief.

- o   Seek supportive workout environments or partners.

8.   Avoid Unhealthy Comparisons:

- o   Focus on your personal progress rather than comparing yourself to others.

- o   Recognize that everyone's fitness journey is unique.

- o   Use others' success as inspiration rather than discouragement.

Remember, overcoming mental barriers is a process. Be patient with yourself and celebrate each step forward, no matter how small it may seem.

3. Building Healthy Habits and Routines

Developing healthy habits is key to long-term fitness success. By turning exercise and healthy behaviors into automatic routines, we reduce the mental effort required to maintain a healthy lifestyle.

The Habit Loop

Understanding the habit loop can help in forming new habits:

1. Cue: A trigger that initiates the behavior.

2. Routine: The behavior itself.

3. Reward: The benefit gained from the behavior.

Strategies for Building Healthy Habits

1. Start Small: Begin with tiny habits that are easy to implement. Example: Do five push-ups every morning after brushing your teeth.

2. Use Habit Stacking: Attach a new habit to an existing one. Example: After pouring your morning coffee, take a 5-minute walk.

3. Make It Easy: Reduce friction for desired habits and increase it for undesired ones. Example: Lay out workout clothes the night before.

4. Be Consistent: Try to perform the habit at the same time each day. Example: Always go for a run at 7 AM.

5. Create a Supportive Environment: Modify your surroundings to support your habits. Example: Keep a yoga mat visible in your living room.

6. Use Visual Cues: Place reminders where you'll see them. Example: Put a "Have you exercised today?" sticky note on your bathroom mirror.

7. Plan for Obstacles: Identify potential barriers and plan how to overcome them. Example: If it's raining, do an indoor workout instead of running outside.

8. Track Your Progress: Use a habit tracker to monitor your consistency. Example: Mark each day you exercise on a calendar.

9. Celebrate Small Wins: Reward yourself for sticking to your habits. Example: After a week of consistent exercise, treat yourself to a movie night.

10. Be Patient: Remember that habit formation takes time, typically 66 days on average.

Creating a Sustainable Fitness Routine

1. Choose Activities You Enjoy: You're more likely to stick with exercises you find fun.

2. Set a Regular Schedule: Consistency is key in forming habits.

3. Balance Different Types of Exercise: Include cardiovascular, strength, and flexibility training.

4. Allow for Rest and Recovery: Build rest days into your routine to prevent burnout.

5. Be Flexible: Have backup plans for when life interferes with your usual routine.

6. Gradually Increase Intensity: Slowly ramp up the challenge to keep progressing and stay engaged.

Remember, the goal is to make fitness a natural part of your daily life, not a chore you dread. Be patient with yourself as you build these new habits and routines.

4. The Role of Self-Efficacy in Fitness Success

Self-efficacy, the belief in one's ability to succeed in specific situations, plays a crucial role in fitness success. High self-efficacy can lead to greater effort and persistence in the face of challenges.

How Self-Efficacy Affects Fitness

1. Goal Setting: People with high self-efficacy set more challenging fitness goals.

2. Effort: Higher self-efficacy leads to greater effort in workouts.

3. Persistence: Those with strong self-efficacy are more likely to stick with their fitness routine despite obstacles.

4.   Resilience: High self-efficacy helps in bouncing back from setbacks.

Sources of Self-Efficacy

1.   Mastery Experiences: Successfully performing a task boosts self-efficacy.

2.   Vicarious Experiences: Seeing others similar to oneself succeed increases belief in one's own abilities.

3.   Verbal Persuasion: Encouragement from others can increase self-efficacy.

4.   Physiological States: How we perceive and interpret our body's responses affects self-efficacy.

Strategies to Boost Self-Efficacy in Fitness

1.   Set Progressive Goals: Start with achievable goals and gradually increase difficulty.

2.   Focus on Process Goals: Emphasize improving skills rather than just outcomes.

3.   Celebrate Small Wins: Acknowledge and celebrate every bit of progress.

4.   Learn Proper Technique: Understanding correct form increases confidence in performing exercises.

5.   Find Role Models: Look for inspiration from people with similar backgrounds who have achieved fitness success.

6.   Seek Positive Feedback: Surround yourself with supportive people who offer constructive encouragement.

7.   Reframe Physiological Responses: Interpret increased heart rate or muscle fatigue as signs of effective exercise rather than distress.

8.   Use Visualization: Imagine yourself successfully completing workouts or achieving fitness goals.

9.   Reflect on Past Successes: Remind yourself of previous fitness achievements, no matter how small.

10. Practice Self-Compassion: Be kind to yourself when facing challenges or setbacks.

Remember, building self-efficacy is a process. Each successful workout or healthy choice builds upon the last, gradually increasing your belief in your ability to achieve your fitness goals.

5. Dealing with Setbacks and Plateaus

Setbacks and plateaus are normal parts of any fitness journey. Learning to navigate these challenges effectively is crucial for long-term success.

Understanding Setbacks and Plateaus

Setbacks: Temporary reversals or interruptions in progress. Examples: Injury, illness, life events disrupting routine.

Plateaus: Periods where progress seems to stall despite continued effort. Examples: Weight loss slowing, strength gains leveling off.

Strategies for Overcoming Setbacks

1. Accept Setbacks as Normal: Understand that setbacks are part of the process, not failures.

2. Identify the Cause: Analyze what led to the setback to prevent future occurrences.

3. Adjust Your Plan: Modify your routine as needed to accommodate the setback.

4. Set Realistic Comeback Goals: Start slowly and gradually build back up to your previous level.

5. Focus on What You Can Do: If injured, work on other aspects of fitness you're able to pursue.

6. Seek Support: Don't hesitate to ask for help from fitness professionals or supportive friends and family.

7. Practice Self-Compassion: Be kind to yourself during the recovery process.

Strategies for Breaking Through Plateaus

1. Vary Your Routine: Introduce new exercises or change the order of your current ones.

2. Adjust Intensity: Increase the weight, reps, or duration of your workouts.

3. Change Frequency: Modify how often you work out or the scheduling of different types of exercise.

4. Focus on Nutrition: Reassess your diet to ensure it's supporting your fitness goals.

5.   Prioritize Recovery: Ensure you're getting adequate rest and sleep.

6.   Set New Goals: Sometimes plateaus indicate it's time to chase new objectives.

7.   Track Different Metrics: Look beyond weight or strength gains to measures like endurance or flexibility.

8.   Seek Expert Advice: Consider working with a trainer to identify areas for improvement.

Remember, setbacks and plateaus are opportunities for learning and growth. Approaching them with a positive, problem-solving mindset can lead to valuable insights and renewed progress.

6. Using Positive Self-Talk and Visualization

The way we talk to ourselves and the images we create in our minds can significantly impact our fitness journey. Positive self-talk and visualization are powerful tools for enhancing motivation, performance, and overall enjoyment of physical activity.

Positive Self-Talk

Self-talk refers to the internal dialogue we have with ourselves. Positive self-talk can boost confidence, reduce anxiety, and improve performance.

Strategies for Positive Self-Talk:

1. Identify Negative Self-Talk: Become aware of negative thoughts or phrases you use. Example: "I can't do this" or "I'm too weak"

2. Challenge Negative Thoughts: Question the validity of negative self-talk. Ask yourself: "Is this really true?" or "What evidence do I have for this thought?"

3. Replace with Positive Affirmations: Substitute negative phrases with positive, encouraging ones. Instead of "This is too hard," try "I can handle this challenge."

4. Use Instructional Self-Talk: Give yourself specific, actionable instructions. Example: "Keep your core tight" or "Focus on your breathing"

5. Develop a Mantra: Create a short, powerful phrase to repeat during challenging moments. Example: "I am strong" or "I've got this"

6. Practice Self-Compassion: Speak to yourself as you would to a good friend. Example: "It's okay to struggle sometimes. You're doing your best."

7. Focus on Effort and Progress: Praise yourself for your hard work and improvements. Example: "I'm proud of myself for showing up today"

Visualization

Visualization involves creating vivid mental images of successfully performing an activity or achieving a goal. This technique can enhance motivation, improve technique, and boost confidence.

How to Use Visualization:

1. Create a Clear Image: Imagine yourself performing your workout or achieving your fitness goal in vivid detail.

2. Engage All Senses: Include not just what you see, but also what you hear, feel, and even smell in your visualization.

3. Visualize Success: Imagine yourself overcoming challenges and succeeding in your fitness endeavors.

4. Practice Regularly: Spend a few minutes each day visualizing your fitness goals and activities.

5. Combine with Relaxation: Use deep breathing or progressive muscle relaxation before visualization to enhance its effectiveness.

6. Use Before Workouts: Visualize a successful workout just before you begin to boost confidence and focus.

7. Visualize the Process: Don't just focus on the end goal; imagine the steps you'll take to get there.

8. Be Realistic: While positive, your visualizations should be grounded in reality to be most effective.

Example Visualization Exercise:

1. Find a quiet, comfortable place to sit or lie down.

2. Take a few deep breaths to relax.

3. Imagine yourself at your next workout. See the gym or outdoor setting in detail.

4.   Picture yourself confidently approaching your exercise equipment.

5.   Visualize yourself performing each exercise with perfect form, feeling strong and capable.

6.   Imagine the satisfaction of completing your workout, feeling energized and proud.

7.   Hold onto this feeling as you open your eyes and return to the present moment.

Remember, both positive self-talk and visualization are skills that improve with practice. Incorporate these techniques into your daily routine to harness their full potential in supporting your fitness journey.

In conclusion, the psychology of fitness plays a crucial role in achieving and maintaining our health and wellness goals. By understanding motivation, overcoming mental barriers, building healthy habits, fostering self-efficacy, dealing with setbacks, and harnessing the power of positive self-talk and visualization, we can create a robust mental framework that supports our physical efforts. Remember, fitness is as much a mental journey as it is a physical one. Cultivating a positive, resilient mindset will not only enhance your fitness outcomes but also contribute to greater overall well-being and life satisfaction.

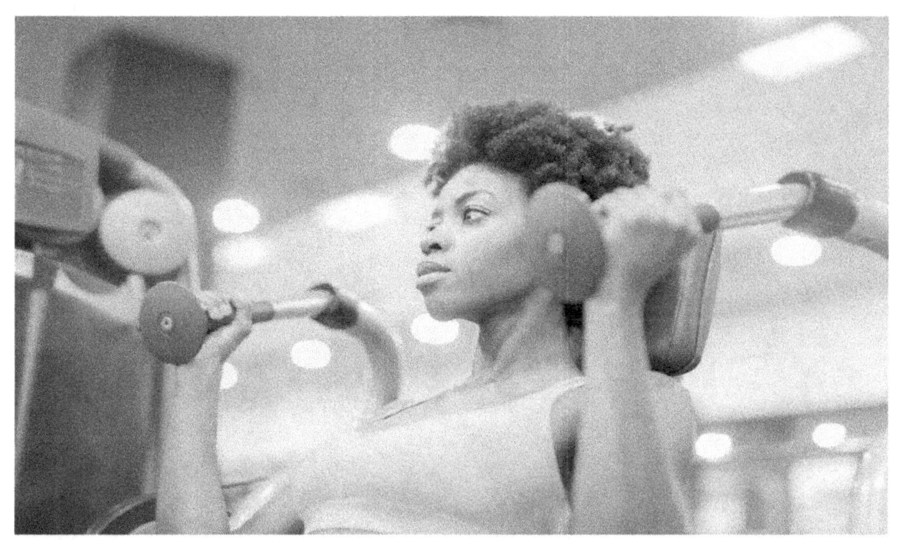

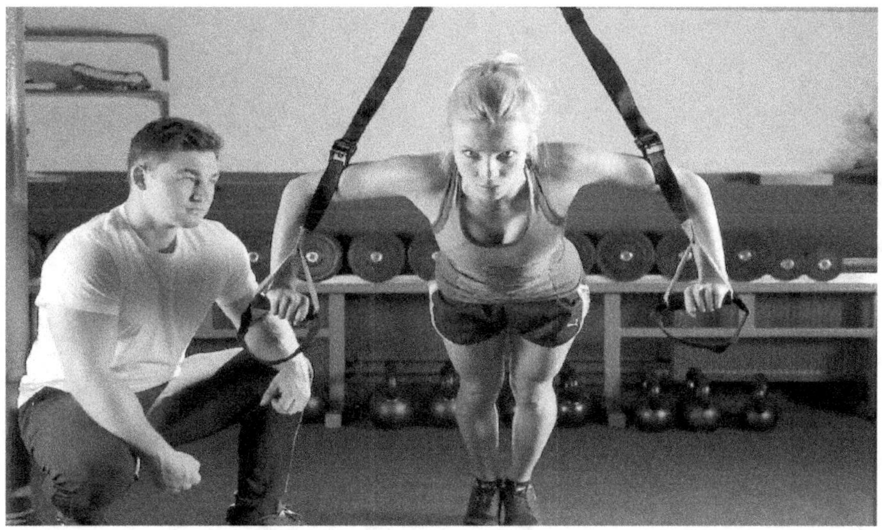

Chapter 8

Technology and Fitness

In recent years, technology has revolutionized the fitness industry, offering new tools and platforms to help individuals achieve their health and wellness goals. This chapter explores the intersection of technology and fitness, discussing various technological advancements and their impact on our fitness journeys.

1. Fitness Apps and Their Effectiveness

Fitness apps have become increasingly popular, offering convenient, personalized ways to track workouts, monitor nutrition, and stay motivated. These apps range from simple step counters to comprehensive fitness ecosystems.

Types of Fitness Apps:

1. Workout Tracking Apps: These apps allow users to log exercises, sets, reps, and weights. Examples: Strong, Fitbod, Jefit.

2. Running and Cycling Apps: Designed for outdoor cardio activities, these apps use GPS to track routes, pace, and distance. Examples: Strava, Nike Run Club, MapMyRun.

3. Nutrition and Diet Apps: These help users track calorie intake, macronutrients, and water consumption. Examples: MyFitnessPal, Lose It!, Noom

4. Yoga and Meditation Apps: Offering guided sessions for mindfulness and flexibility. Examples: Yoga Studio, Headspace, Calm

5. All-in-One Fitness Apps: Comprehensive platforms that combine workout tracking, nutrition, and sometimes community features. Examples: MyFitnessPal, Fitbit App, Apple Health

Effectiveness of Fitness Apps:

Research has shown that fitness apps can be effective tools for improving health and fitness outcomes when used consistently. Some key benefits include:

1. Increased Awareness: Apps help users become more conscious of their activity levels, nutrition, and progress.

2. Goal Setting and Tracking: Many apps allow users to set specific goals and track progress over time, which can boost motivation.

3. Personalization: Advanced apps use algorithms to tailor workouts and nutrition plans to individual needs and preferences.

4.   Convenience: Apps make it easy to access workout plans, nutrition information, and tracking tools anytime, anywhere.

5.   Education: Many apps provide educational content about exercise techniques, nutrition, and general health.

6.   Motivation: Features like achievements, streaks, and social sharing can help keep users motivated.

However, the effectiveness of fitness apps largely depends on user engagement. To maximize the benefits:

1.   Choose an app that aligns with your specific fitness goals.

2.   Be consistent in using the app to track your activities.

3.   Take advantage of educational resources within the app.

4.   Use the app's community features for added support and motivation.

5.   Regularly review your progress and adjust goals as needed.

Remember, while fitness apps can be powerful tools, they should complement, not replace, professional guidance when necessary.

2. Wearable Technology for Tracking Progress

Wearable fitness technology has evolved from simple pedometers to sophisticated devices that can monitor various aspects of health and fitness. These devices offer real-time data and insights to help users optimize their fitness routines.

Common Types of Fitness Wearables:

1.   Fitness Trackers: Basic devices that monitor steps, distance, calories burned, and sometimes sleep. Examples: Fitbit Charge, Garmin Vivosmart

2.   Smartwatches: More advanced devices that combine fitness tracking with smartwatch features like notifications and apps. Examples: Apple Watch, Samsung Galaxy Watch

3.   Heart Rate Monitors: Devices specifically designed to track heart rate during exercise. Examples: Polar H10, Wahoo TICKR

4.   Smart Clothing: Garments with embedded sensors to track various metrics. Examples: Athos Training System, Hexoskin Smart Shirts

Key Metrics Tracked by Wearables:

1.   Steps and Distance: Basic measure of daily activity.

2.   Heart Rate: Helps gauge exercise intensity and overall cardiovascular health.

3.   Calories Burned: Estimates energy expenditure throughout the day.

4.   Sleep Patterns: Monitors duration and quality of sleep.

5.   VO2 Max: Some advanced devices estimate this measure of cardiorespiratory fitness.

6.   Stress Levels: Often measured through heart rate variability.

7.   Blood Oxygen Levels: Some devices can measure SpO2 levels.

Benefits of Using Wearables:

1.   Continuous Monitoring: Provides a comprehensive view of daily activity and health metrics.

2.   Motivation: Visual representations of progress can encourage users to stay active.

3.   Goal Setting: Many devices allow users to set and track specific fitness goals.

4.   Workout Optimization: Real-time data can help users adjust workout intensity.

5.   Sleep Insights: Sleep tracking can help users improve sleep habits.

6.   Integration with Apps: Many wearables sync with fitness apps for a more comprehensive view of health data.

Considerations When Using Wearables:

1.   Accuracy: While generally reliable, wearables may not be as accurate as medical-grade devices.

2.   Privacy: Consider the privacy implications of sharing health data with device manufacturers.

3.   Dependency: Be cautious about becoming overly reliant on devices for motivation.

4.   Overemphasis on Data: Remember that numbers don't tell the whole story of health and fitness.

145 | Technology and Fitness

To effectively use wearables for tracking progress:

1. Set realistic goals based on your current fitness level.

2. Use the data to identify patterns and areas for improvement.

3. Regularly review your progress and adjust your fitness plan accordingly.

4. Don't obsess over daily fluctuations; focus on long-term trends.

5. Use the insights gained to have more informed discussions with fitness professionals or healthcare providers.

3. Virtual Fitness Classes and Online Coaching

The rise of virtual fitness classes and online coaching has made expert guidance and group workouts more accessible than ever. These digital alternatives to traditional gym classes and personal training offer flexibility and variety to fit diverse lifestyles and preferences.

Virtual Fitness Classes:

Types of Virtual Classes:

1. Live-streamed Classes: Real-time sessions led by instructors, often allowing for interaction.

2. On-demand Classes: Pre-recorded sessions that can be accessed anytime.

3. Interactive Classes: Sessions that use technology to provide real-time feedback, often through connected equipment.

Popular Platforms:

- Peloton
- Les Mills On Demand
- Beachbody On Demand
- Alo Moves (for yoga)
- Zwift (for cycling and running)

Benefits of Virtual Classes:

1. Convenience: Work out anytime, anywhere.

2. Variety: Access to a wide range of class types and instructors.

3. Cost-effective: Often cheaper than gym memberships or in-person classes.

4. Privacy: Ideal for those who feel self-conscious in group settings.

5. Consistency: Makes it easier to maintain a regular workout schedule.

Online Coaching:

Types of Online Coaching:

1. One-on-one Video Coaching: Personal training sessions conducted via video call.

2. Programmed Workouts: Customized workout plans delivered through apps or email.

3. Form Check and Feedback: Coaches review videos of exercises and provide feedback.

4. Nutrition Coaching: Guidance on diet and nutrition to complement fitness goals.

Benefits of Online Coaching:

1. Personalization: Workouts and advice tailored to individual needs and goals.

2. Flexibility: Communicate with coaches on your schedule.

3. Accountability: Regular check-ins help keep you on track.

4. Access to Expertise: Work with specialized coaches regardless of location.

5. Cost-effective: Often more affordable than in-person personal training.

Making the Most of Virtual Fitness:

1. Create a dedicated workout space at home.

2. Invest in basic equipment for a variety of workouts.

3. Schedule your virtual workouts like you would in-person classes.

4. Engage with the community features of your chosen platform.

5. Communicate openly with online coaches about your progress and challenges.

6. Mix live and on-demand classes to balance structure and flexibility.

While virtual fitness options offer many advantages, they may not be suitable for everyone. Consider your personal preferences, motivation levels, and any health considerations when deciding between virtual and in-person fitness options.

4. Social Media and Fitness Communities

Social media has become a significant influencer in the fitness world, creating virtual communities where individuals can share experiences, seek advice, and find motivation. These platforms have transformed how people approach fitness, offering both opportunities and challenges.

Popular Social Media Platforms for Fitness:

1. Instagram: Known for fitness influencers, transformation photos, and workout videos.

2. YouTube: Home to countless fitness channels offering workout videos and educational content.

3. Facebook Groups: Communities centered around specific fitness interests or programs.

4. Reddit: Subreddits dedicated to various aspects of fitness, from weightlifting to nutrition.

5. TikTok: Short-form videos featuring workout tips, challenges, and transformations.

Benefits of Fitness Social Media:

1.   Inspiration: Success stories and transformation photos can be motivating.

2.   Education: Access to free workout ideas, nutrition tips, and fitness information.

3.   Community Support: Connecting with like-minded individuals for encouragement and advice.

4.   Accountability: Sharing goals and progress can help maintain commitment.

5.   Diversity: Exposure to various fitness approaches and body types.

Challenges of Fitness Social Media:

1.   Misinformation: Not all advice shared on social media is accurate or safe.

2.   Unrealistic Expectations: Carefully curated posts may not represent realistic outcomes.

3.   Comparison Trap: Constantly comparing oneself to others can be demotivating.

4.   Overemphasis on Aesthetics: Some content may prioritize appearance over health.

5.   Information Overload: The sheer volume of content can be overwhelming.

Using Social Media Effectively for Fitness:

1.   Curate Your Feed: Follow accounts that genuinely inspire and educate you.

2.   Fact-Check Information: Verify fitness advice with reputable sources.

3.   Set Boundaries: Limit social media time to avoid negative impacts on mental health.

4.   Engage Mindfully: Participate in communities that align with your values and goals.

5.   Share Responsibly: If you post about your fitness journey, be honest about your experiences.

6.   Remember Individual Differences: What works for one person may not work for everyone.

7.   Use as a Tool, Not a Replacement: Social media should complement, not replace, professional guidance.

Online Fitness Communities: Many platforms host dedicated fitness communities that offer more focused interactions:

1.   Strava: A social network for athletes, particularly popular among runners and cyclists.

2.   MyFitnessPal Forums: Discussions on various topics related to nutrition and fitness.

3.   Fitbit Community: Users of Fitbit devices share experiences and challenges.

4.   Bodybuilding.com BodySpace: A social network specifically for strength training enthusiasts.

These communities can provide valuable support, but it's important to approach them with a critical mind and always prioritize your individual health and well-being.

5. The Pros and Cons of Tech-Driven Fitness

As technology becomes increasingly integrated into our fitness routines, it's important to consider both its advantages and potential drawbacks.

Pros of Tech-Driven Fitness:

1. Accessibility: Technology makes fitness information and guidance more widely available.

2. Personalization: Apps and devices can tailor workouts and nutrition plans to individual needs.

3. Tracking and Data: Detailed metrics allow for more informed decision-making about fitness strategies.

4. Motivation: Gamification elements and social features can boost engagement and consistency.

5. Convenience: Virtual classes and on-demand content make it easier to fit fitness into busy schedules.

6. Education: Many tech tools provide in-depth information about exercise techniques and health topics.

7. Community: Online platforms facilitate connections with like-minded individuals for support and inspiration.

8. Cost-Effectiveness: Many tech solutions are more affordable than traditional gym memberships or personal training.

Cons of Tech-Driven Fitness:

1. Over-reliance on Technology: Dependency on devices or apps may diminish intrinsic motivation.

2. Data Accuracy Concerns: Consumer-grade devices may not always provide medical-grade accuracy.

3. Privacy Issues: Sharing personal health data raises questions about data security and use.

4. Information Overload: The abundance of available information can be overwhelming and sometimes contradictory.

5. Reduced Human Interaction: Overuse of tech may limit valuable in-person coaching and community experiences.

6. Distraction: Constant checking of devices or social media can detract from the workout experience.

7. Comparison and Self-Esteem Issues: Exposure to idealized body images and achievements on social media can negatively impact self-esteem.

8. Technical Barriers: Not everyone has equal access to or comfort with using fitness technology.

6. Balancing Technology Use with Mindful Exercise

While technology offers numerous benefits for fitness, it's crucial to find a balance that enhances rather than detracts from the exercise experience. Mindful exercise involves being fully present during your workout, aware of your body's movements and sensations.

Strategies for Balancing Tech Use and Mindful Exercise:

1. Designated Tech-Free Workouts: Set aside some sessions where you exercise without any technology, focusing solely on your body and the present moment.

2. Limit Checking Devices: If using a fitness tracker, resist the urge to constantly check it during your workout. Set specific times to review your data.

3. Mindful Warm-Up and Cool-Down: Use the beginning and end of your workout as tech-free times to connect with your body.

4. Intentional Tech Use: When you do use technology during workouts, be clear about its purpose (e.g., for tracking, guidance, or motivation).

5. Practice Bodyweight Exercises: Incorporate exercises that require no equipment, allowing you to focus on form and mind-muscle connection.

6. Outdoor Workouts: Spend time exercising in nature without headphones, engaging with your environment.

7. Mindfulness Apps: Paradoxically, some apps can help cultivate mindfulness. Use guided meditations or body scans before or after workouts.

8. Reflect Without Tech: After workouts, take a few minutes to mentally review how you feel, rather than immediately checking your stats.

9. Social Media Boundaries: Set specific times for engaging with fitness social media, separate from your actual workout times.

10. Listen to Your Body: Learn to tune into your body's signals without relying solely on tech-based data.

Finding Your Balance: The ideal balance between technology use and mindful exercise will vary for each individual. Experiment with different approaches to find what works best for you. Remember, technology should enhance your fitness journey, not dominate it.

Technology has undoubtedly transformed the fitness landscape, offering powerful tools for tracking, motivation, and education. From fitness apps and wearables to virtual classes and online communities, tech-driven fitness solutions provide unprecedented access to resources that can support our health and wellness goals.

However, it's crucial to approach these technologies mindfully. While they offer numerous benefits, over-reliance on tech can sometimes disconnect us from the inherent joy and mindfulness of physical activity. The key is to harness the benefits of fitness technology while maintaining a balanced, mindful approach to exercise. Distinguish between the discomfort of pushing your limits and actual pain that could indicate harm.

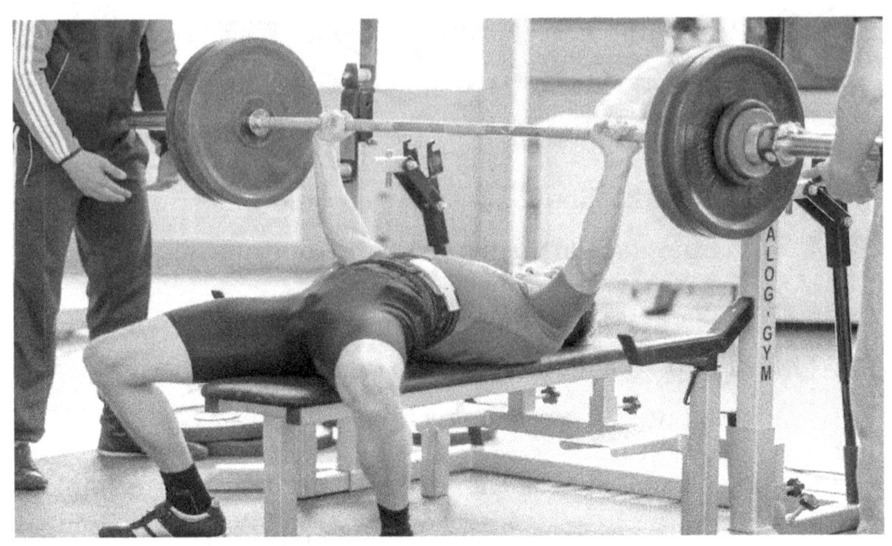

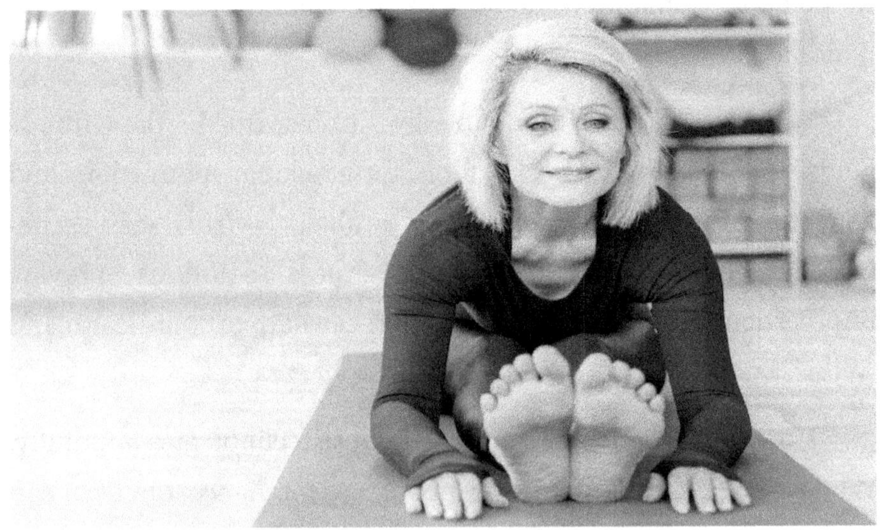

Chapter 9

Nutrition and Fitness Myths Debunked

In the world of health and fitness, myths and misconceptions abound. These false beliefs can lead to ineffective strategies, wasted effort, and even potential harm. This chapter aims to debunk common myths surrounding nutrition and fitness, providing evidence-based information to help you make informed decisions about your health.

1. Common Misconceptions About Diet and Exercise

Let's start by addressing some of the most prevalent myths about diet and exercise:

Myth: "No pain, no gain"

Reality: While challenging yourself is important, pain is not a necessary part of an effective workout. In fact, pain often signals potential injury. It's crucial to distinguish between the discomfort of pushing your limits and actual pain that could indicate harm.

Myth: "You need to eat every 2-3 hours to boost metabolism"

Reality: Meal frequency has little effect on metabolism. What matters most is total daily calorie intake. Some people may prefer frequent small meals, while others do well with fewer, larger meals. Choose an eating pattern that fits your lifestyle and helps you maintain a balanced diet.

Myth: "Carbs are bad for you"

Reality: Carbohydrates are a crucial macronutrient. The key is choosing complex carbs (whole grains, fruits, vegetables) over simple carbs (sugary snacks, white bread). Carbs provide energy for your body and brain, and are especially important for high-intensity exercise.

Myth: "Fat makes you fat"

Reality: Dietary fat doesn't directly translate to body fat. Fats are essential for hormone production, nutrient absorption, and cell health. Excessive calorie intake from any source (fat, carbs, or protein) can lead to weight gain. Healthy fats (like those in avocados, nuts, and olive oil) should be part of a balanced diet.

Myth: "You need to do cardio to lose weight"

Reality: While cardiovascular exercise is beneficial for heart health and can aid in creating a calorie deficit, it's not the only way to lose weight. A combination of strength training and a balanced diet can be equally, if not more, effective for weight loss and overall health.

Myth: "Eating late at night causes weight gain"

Reality: When you eat doesn't matter as much as what and how much you eat. Total daily calorie intake is the primary factor in weight gain or loss. However, late-night eating might lead to consuming extra calories if it's in addition to, rather than part of, your regular meals.

Myth: "Detox diets cleanse your body of toxins"

Reality: Your liver and kidneys are highly efficient at removing toxins from your body. There's no scientific evidence that detox diets or cleanses remove toxins better than these organs. A balanced diet rich in fruits, vegetables, and water supports your body's natural detoxification processes.

Myth: "You need to drink 8 glasses of water a day"

Reality: While staying hydrated is crucial, there's no one-size-fits-all rule for water intake. Your needs depend on factors like activity level, climate, and diet. Many foods also contribute to your daily fluid intake. Listen to your body and drink when you're thirsty.

Understanding these realities can help you make more informed decisions about your diet and exercise routine, leading to more effective and sustainable health practices.

2. The Truth About Fad Diets and Quick Fixes

Fad diets and quick-fix solutions are perennially popular, promising rapid weight loss or dramatic health improvements.

However, these approaches often fail to deliver long-term results and can sometimes be harmful.

Common Types of Fad Diets:

1. Extreme Calorie Restriction: Diets that severely limit calorie intake.

2. Food Group Elimination: Diets that completely cut out entire food groups.

3. "Detox" or "Cleanse" Diets: Short-term diets claiming to rid the body of toxins.

4. "Miracle Food" Diets: Diets centered around consuming large amounts of a single food.

5. Liquid Diets: Replacing most or all solid foods with juices or shakes.

The Reality of Fad Diets:

1. Short-Term Results: Many fad diets lead to quick initial weight loss, often due to water loss or severe calorie restriction. However, this weight is usually regained once normal eating resumes.

2. Nutrient Deficiencies: Extreme diets often lack essential nutrients, potentially leading to health issues over time.

3. Metabolic Slowdown: Severe calorie restriction can slow metabolism, making it harder to maintain weight loss in the long term.

4. Unsustainable: Most fad diets are difficult to maintain long-term, leading to a cycle of weight loss and regain known as "yo-yo dieting."

5. Potential Health Risks: Some extreme diets can lead to electrolyte imbalances, dehydration, or other health complications.

6. Ignores Individual Needs: Fad diets often take a one-size-fits-all approach, ignoring individual nutritional needs and preferences.

The Truth About Quick Fixes:

1. "Fat-Burning" Pills: Most of these supplements have minimal effect on weight loss and can have side effects.

2. "Waist Trainers" or "Sweat Belts": These don't cause fat loss in specific areas; they may temporarily reduce water weight but can also restrict breathing and movement.

3. Extreme Exercise Regimens: While exercise is crucial for health, extreme programs can lead to burnout or injury, especially for beginners.

4. "Negative Calorie" Foods: No food has negative calories. While some foods (like celery) are very low in calories, they don't cause the body to burn more calories than they contain.

The Sustainable Approach:

Instead of falling for fad diets or quick fixes, focus on sustainable lifestyle changes:

1.   Balanced Diet: Eat a variety of foods from all food groups, focusing on whole, minimally processed options.

2.   Moderate Calorie Reduction: For weight loss, aim for a modest calorie deficit (about 500 calories per day) rather than extreme restriction.

3.   Regular Physical Activity: Incorporate both cardio and strength training into your routine.

4.   Mindful Eating: Pay attention to hunger and fullness cues, and eat without distractions.

5.   Gradual Changes: Make small, sustainable changes to your diet and exercise habits over time.

6.   Personalization: Work with a registered dietitian or nutritionist to create a plan tailored to your individual needs and goals.

Remember, healthy weight loss and improved fitness take time. Be patient with your body and focus on building habits you can maintain for life.

3. Separating Fact from Fiction in Supplement Claims

The supplement industry is rife with bold claims and promises of miraculous results. While some supplements can be beneficial, many are unnecessary for most people, and some can even be harmful. Here's how to navigate supplement claims:

Common Supplement Myths:

1. "This supplement melts fat away" Reality: No supplement can directly cause fat loss. Weight loss occurs when you consume fewer calories than you burn.

2. "This product builds muscle instantly" Reality: Muscle growth requires consistent strength training and adequate protein intake. No supplement can replace this process.

3. "This herb cures [insert health condition]" Reality: While some herbs have medicinal properties, claims of "cures" are often exaggerated. Always consult a healthcare provider for medical conditions.

4. "This supplement is all-natural, so it's completely safe" Reality: "Natural" doesn't always mean safe. Many potent drugs are derived from natural sources. Some natural supplements can interact with medications or have side effects.

5. "This vitamin boosts your immune system" Reality: While certain nutrients are important for immune function, taking extra vitamins beyond what your body needs doesn't "boost" immunity for most healthy people.

How to Evaluate Supplement Claims:

1. Look for Scientific Evidence: Reputable supplements should have peer-reviewed research supporting their claims.

2. Check for Third-Party Testing: Organizations like NSF International or USP verify the content and purity of supplements.

3.   Be Wary of Anecdotal Evidence: Personal testimonials are not scientific proof of a supplement's effectiveness.

4.   Understand Regulation: In many countries, supplements are not strictly regulated. Claims may not be verified by regulatory bodies.

5.   Consult Professionals: Talk to a doctor or registered dietitian before starting any new supplement regimen.

Supplements That May Have Benefits (for some people):

1.   Vitamin D: For those with limited sun exposure or deficiency.

2.   Omega-3 Fatty Acids: Particularly for those who don't eat fatty fish regularly.

3.   Probiotics: May help with digestive issues in some people.

4.   Protein Supplements: Can be useful for athletes or those struggling to get enough protein from food.

5.   Creatine: Has been shown to enhance performance in high-intensity, short-duration activities.

Remember, for most people, a balanced diet provides all necessary nutrients. Supplements should supplement, not replace, a healthy diet.

4. Understanding the Limitations of BMI

Body Mass Index (BMI) is a widely used measure to categorize individuals as underweight, normal weight, overweight, or obese. However, it has significant limitations that are often overlooked.

What is BMI?

BMI is calculated by dividing a person's weight in kilograms by their height in meters squared (kg/m^2). The resulting number is then categorized:

- Underweight: Less than 18.5

- Normal weight: 18.5 to 24.9

- Overweight: 25 to 29.9

- Obese: 30 or greater

Limitations of BMI:

1. Doesn't Distinguish Between Fat and Muscle: BMI doesn't differentiate between body fat and lean mass. Athletes or muscular individuals may be classified as overweight or obese despite having low body fat.

2. Ignores Body Composition: Two people with the same BMI can have very different body compositions and health risks.

3. Doesn't Account for Fat Distribution: Where fat is stored in the body (e.g., abdominal vs. hip area) can be more indicative of health risks than total body fat.

4. Age and Gender Differences: BMI doesn't account for natural changes in body composition that occur with age or differences between genders.

5. Ethnic Variations: BMI thresholds may not be appropriate for all ethnic groups. For example, some Asian populations may have increased health risks at lower BMI levels.

6. Height Extremes: BMI may overestimate body fat in very tall individuals and underestimate it in very short individuals.

Alternative Measures:

1. Waist Circumference: Can be a better indicator of abdominal fat, which is associated with higher health risks.

2. Waist-to-Hip Ratio: Another measure of fat distribution that can indicate health risks.

3. Body Fat Percentage: Directly measures the proportion of fat in the body. Can be assessed through methods like skinfold measurements, bioelectrical impedance, or DEXA scans.

4. ABSI (A Body Shape Index): Considers waist circumference in relation to height and weight.

5. Fitness Level: Cardiovascular fitness and strength can be more indicative of overall health than BMI alone.

While BMI can be a useful screening tool at a population level, it should not be the sole determinant of an individual's health status. A comprehensive assessment should include other measures, lifestyle factors, and individual health history.

5. The Myth of Spot Reduction

Spot reduction refers to the belief that you can target fat loss in specific areas of your body through particular exercises. This is one of the most persistent myths in fitness.

The Myth:

The idea behind spot reduction is that by exercising a specific body part, you can burn fat in that area. For example, doing lots of crunches to lose belly fat or tricep exercises to get rid of arm fat.

The Reality:

1. Fat Loss is Systemic: When you burn fat, it comes from all over your body, not just the area you're exercising.

2. Genetics Play a Role: Where you lose fat first is largely determined by your genetics and hormones.

3. Muscle Building vs. Fat Loss: While you can build muscle in specific areas, you can't target fat loss in the same way.

4. Overall Calorie Deficit is Key: Fat loss occurs when you're in a calorie deficit, regardless of what exercises you're doing.

Why the Myth Persists:

1. Muscle Tone: Exercises for specific body parts can increase muscle tone, which might create the appearance of fat loss.

2. Temporary Swelling: Working out a specific area can cause temporary swelling, making that area appear smaller.

3. Marketing: Many products and programs are sold based on the promise of spot reduction.

Effective Approaches for Fat Loss:

1. Full-Body Strength Training: Building muscle all over your body increases metabolism.

2. Cardiovascular Exercise: Helps create a calorie deficit and improves overall health.

3. Balanced Diet: Focus on whole foods and appropriate portion sizes.

4. Consistency: Regular exercise and healthy eating habits over time lead to overall fat loss.

5. Patience: Different areas of your body may lose fat at different rates. Be patient and consistent.

Remember, while you can't spot reduce, you can spot strengthen. Building muscle in specific areas can help shape your body and improve overall body composition.

6. Addressing Gender-Specific Fitness Myths

Many fitness myths are specifically targeted at or perpetuated among certain genders. Let's address some common gender-specific fitness myths:

Myths Often Targeted at Women:

1.   Myth: "Lifting weights will make women bulky" Reality:
     Women typically don't have enough testosterone to build
     large muscles without specific training and dietary
     protocols. Weight training helps women build lean muscle,
     increase metabolism, and achieve a toned appearance.

2.   Myth: "Women should stick to light weights and high reps
     for toning" Reality: Challenging weights are necessary for
     muscle development and strength gains. "Toning" is
     actually a combination of muscle building and fat loss.

3.   Myth: "Women shouldn't exercise during pregnancy"
     Reality: In most cases, exercise during pregnancy is safe and
     beneficial. However, it's important to consult with a
     healthcare provider and modify activities as needed.

4.   Myth: "The thigh gap is a sign of fitness" Reality: Thigh gaps
     are largely determined by bone structure and genetics, not
     fitness level. Focusing on overall health and strength is more
     important than arbitrary aesthetic standards.

Myths Often Targeted at Men:

1.   Myth: "Men don't need to worry about osteoporosis"
     Reality: While less common than in women, men can
     develop osteoporosis. Weight-bearing exercises and
     adequate calcium and vitamin D are important for bone
     health in both genders.

2.   Myth: "Cardio will make you lose muscle" Reality: While
     excessive cardio combined with inadequate nutrition can
     lead to muscle loss, moderate cardio can improve overall

fitness without significant muscle loss, especially when combined with strength training and proper nutrition.

3. Myth: "Men should focus on upper body and skip leg day" Reality: A balanced workout routine that includes lower body exercises is crucial for overall strength, athleticism, and injury prevention.

4. Myth: "Protein shakes are necessary for muscle growth" Reality: While protein is important for muscle building, most men can get adequate protein through a balanced diet. Supplements can be convenient but aren't necessary for everyone.

Gender-Neutral Fitness Truths:

1. Consistency is Key: Regular exercise is more important than intense but infrequent workouts.

2. Nutrition Matters: You can't out-exercise a poor diet. Balanced nutrition is crucial for both men and women.

3. Rest and Recovery are Important: Adequate sleep and rest days are essential for progress and injury prevention.

4. Individual Variations Exist: What works for one person may not work for another, regardless of gender.

5. Health Goes Beyond Appearance: Focus on how you feel and what your body can do, not just how it looks.

6. Strength Training is Beneficial for Everyone: Both men and women can benefit from resistance training for health, functionality, and body composition.

7.   Flexibility and Mobility Matter: Incorporate stretching and mobility work into your routine, regardless of gender.

By debunking these gender-specific myths, we can promote a more inclusive and accurate understanding of fitness that benefits everyone. Remember, the principles of exercise science apply to all genders, even if individual responses may vary.

In the world of nutrition and fitness, myths and misconceptions can lead us astray from our health goals. By understanding the facts behind common myths about diet, exercise, supplements, body measurements, fat loss, and gender-specific fitness beliefs, we can make more informed decisions about our health and wellness practices.

Remember that the field of health and fitness is constantly evolving as new research emerges. What we consider fact today may be challenged or refined tomorrow. This is why it's crucial to:

1.   Stay Informed: Keep up with reputable health and fitness sources, but be critical of sensational claims.

2.   Consult Professionals: Work with certified fitness trainers, registered dietitians, and healthcare providers for personalized advice.

3.   Listen to Your Body: Pay attention to how different foods and exercises make you feel. Everyone's body responds differently.

4.   Focus on Sustainable Practices: Instead of quick fixes, prioritize habits you can maintain long-term.

5.   Be Wary of Extremes: If a claim or approach seems too good to be true or unnecessarily restrictive, it probably is.

6.   Understand Individual Variation: What works for one person may not work for another. Be patient in finding what works best for you.

7.   Prioritize Overall Health: Remember that health encompasses physical, mental, and emotional well-being, not just appearance or performance.

By debunking these myths, we hope to empower you with knowledge that supports a balanced, sustainable approach to health and fitness. As you continue your wellness journey, maintain a curious and critical mindset. Question bold claims, seek evidence-based information, and remember that true health is a lifelong journey, not a destination reached through quick fixes or extreme measures.

Ultimately, the most effective approach to nutrition and fitness is one that you can maintain consistently, that makes you feel good both physically and mentally, and that aligns with your personal health goals and values.

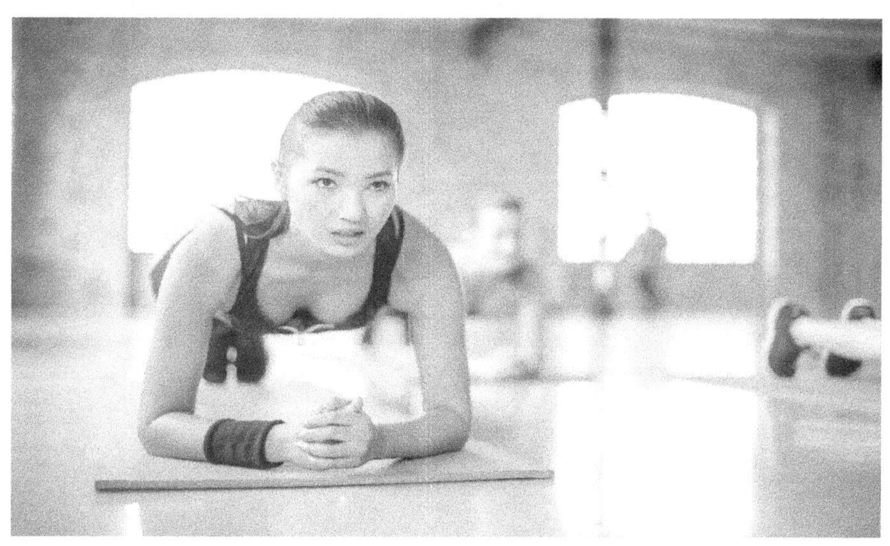

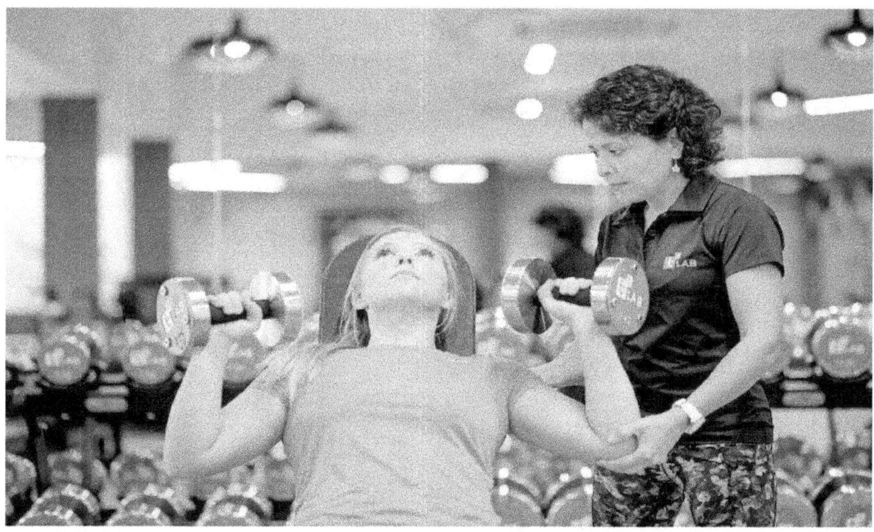

Chapter 10

Long-term Success and Lifestyle Integration

Achieving fitness goals is one thing but maintaining them for the long haul is another challenge entirely. This chapter focuses on strategies to integrate healthy habits into your lifestyle for lasting success, ensuring that your fitness journey becomes a sustainable part of your life rather than a temporary phase.

1. Transitioning from 'Dieting' to Lifestyle Change

The concept of 'dieting' often implies a temporary change in eating habits, usually with the goal of losing weight. However, for long-term success, it's crucial to shift from this mindset to one of permanent lifestyle change.

Problems with the 'Dieting' Mentality:

1. Temporary Nature: Diets are often seen as short-term solutions, leading to a cycle of weight loss and regain.

2.   Restrictive Approach: Many diets involve cutting out entire food groups or severely limiting calories, which is often unsustainable.

3.   All-or-Nothing Thinking: The dieting mindset can lead to feelings of failure if you don't stick to the plan perfectly.

4.   Neglect of Other Health Factors: Diets often focus solely on weight loss, ignoring other aspects of health like nutrition, mental wellbeing, and physical fitness.

Shifting to a Lifestyle Change Approach:

1.   Focus on Whole Foods: Instead of following strict diet rules, emphasize consuming a variety of whole, nutrient-dense foods.

2.   Practice Mindful Eating: Pay attention to hunger and fullness cues, eat slowly, and enjoy your food without guilt.

3.   Cook More Often: Preparing your own meals gives you control over ingredients and portion sizes.

4.   Make Gradual Changes: Instead of overhauling your entire diet at once, make small, sustainable changes over time.

5.   Allow for Flexibility: Include all foods in moderation, without labeling them as 'good' or 'bad'.

6.   Prioritize Nutrient Density: Focus on getting the most nutritional bang for your caloric buck, rather than just counting calories.

7. Consider Long-Term Health: Make food choices based on how they contribute to your overall health and wellbeing, not just short-term weight loss.

8. Integrate Physical Activity: View exercise as a regular part of your routine, not just a weight loss tool.

9. Develop a Healthy Relationship with Food: Work on eliminating guilt and anxiety around eating.

10. Seek Support: Surround yourself with people who support your healthy lifestyle changes.

Remember, the goal is to create habits that you can maintain for life, not just until you reach a certain number on the scale. This approach leads to better health outcomes and a more positive relationship with food and your body.

2. Strategies for Maintaining Motivation

Motivation can fluctuate over time, especially when pursuing long-term goals. Here are strategies to help maintain your motivation for a healthy lifestyle:

1. Set Meaningful Goals: Ensure your fitness goals align with your values and what truly matters to you. This intrinsic motivation is more powerful than external factors.

2. Break Down Large Goals: Divide big goals into smaller, manageable milestones. This provides regular sense of achievement and progress.

3. Track Progress: Keep a record of your workouts, meals, or how you feel. Seeing progress, even small improvements, can be highly motivating.

4. Reward Yourself: Set up a reward system for reaching milestones. Make sure the rewards don't contradict your health goals.

5. Visualize Success: Regularly imagine yourself achieving your goals. Visualization can boost motivation and confidence.

6. Find Your 'Why': Regularly remind yourself why you started this journey. Connect with your deeper reasons for pursuing a healthy lifestyle.

7. Create a Support System: Surround yourself with supportive people. Consider joining fitness classes or online communities for added motivation.

8. Mix It Up: Avoid boredom by trying new workouts, recipes, or fitness challenges. Variety can reignite motivation.

9. Schedule Your Workouts: Treat exercise like any other important appointment. Having a set schedule can help maintain consistency.

10. Focus on Feeling Good: Pay attention to how exercise and healthy eating make you feel. The positive feelings can be a powerful motivator.

11. Use Positive Self-Talk: Be your own cheerleader. Practice encouraging self-talk, especially when facing challenges.

12. Learn Continuously: Educate yourself about health and fitness. Understanding the 'why' behind healthy habits can increase motivation to maintain them.

13. Prepare for Setbacks: Recognize that setbacks are normal. Have a plan for how you'll get back on track when they occur.

14. Celebrate Non-Scale Victories: Acknowledge improvements in energy, mood, sleep, or fitness level, not just changes in weight.

15. Make it Social: Exercise with friends or join group activities. Social connections can make fitness more enjoyable and motivating.

Remember, motivation is not a constant state. It's normal for it to ebb and flow. The key is to have multiple strategies you can rely on to keep you moving forward, even when motivation is low.

3. Adapting Your Fitness Routine to Life Changes

Life is full of changes - career shifts, relationships, family responsibilities, health issues, and more. A sustainable fitness routine should be flexible enough to adapt to these changes while still supporting your health goals.

Common Life Changes and Adaptation Strategies:

1. New Job or Changed Work Hours:

     o   Reassess your schedule and find new time slots for exercise.

- o Consider shorter, more intense workouts if time is limited.

   - o Explore lunch-break workouts or active commuting options.

2. Relationship Changes:

   - o Involve your partner in your fitness routine.

   - o Find activities you both enjoy to make fitness a shared experience.

   - o Communicate the importance of your health goals to your partner.

3. Becoming a Parent:

   - o Explore workouts you can do with your baby (like jogging with a stroller).

   - o Use nap times for quick home workouts.

   - o Consider family-friendly activities like hiking or swimming.

4. Injury or Health Issues:

   - o Work with healthcare providers to modify your routine safely.

   - o Focus on exercises that support recovery and overall health.

   - o Use this time to explore new, low-impact activities like yoga or swimming.

5.   Relocation:

- o   Research fitness options in your new area.

- o   Use this as an opportunity to try new outdoor activities or local sports.

- o   Set up a home gym if access to fitness facilities is limited.

6.   Increased Work or Family Responsibilities:

- o   Break workouts into shorter sessions throughout the day.

- o   Prioritize efficiency with HIIT or circuit training.

- o   Integrate movement into daily tasks (like squats while brushing teeth).

7.   Financial Changes:

- o   Explore free workout resources online or in your community.

- o   Invest in basic home equipment for cost-effective, long-term fitness.

- o   Consider bodyweight exercises that require no equipment.

8.   Aging:

- o   Gradually modify your routine to include more joint-friendly exercises.

- o   Increase focus on balance and flexibility work.

- o   Consult with fitness professionals who specialize in training older adults.

General Principles for Adapting Your Fitness Routine:

1. Be Flexible: Have multiple workout options of varying durations and intensities.

2. Prioritize Consistency Over Perfection: Some exercise is always better than none.

3. Reassess Regularly: Review your routine every few months or after major life changes.

4. Focus on Habits, Not Just Workouts: Look for ways to increase daily movement, not just structured exercise.

5. Embrace New Challenges: View life changes as opportunities to diversify your fitness experiences.

Remember, a fitness routine that can adapt to life's changes is one you're more likely to maintain long-term. The goal is to make fitness a consistent part of your life, regardless of what changes come your way.

4. The Importance of Rest and Recovery

In the pursuit of fitness goals, the importance of rest and recovery is often overlooked. However, these elements are crucial for long-term success, injury prevention, and overall wellbeing.

Why Rest and Recovery Matter:

1. Muscle Repair and Growth: Exercise creates micro-tears in muscle fibers. Rest allows these fibers to repair and grow stronger.

2. Prevent Overtraining: Continuous intense exercise without adequate rest can lead to overtraining syndrome, resulting in decreased performance and increased injury risk.

3. Mental Refreshment: Rest days provide a mental break, helping prevent burnout and maintain motivation.

4. Hormonal Balance: Proper recovery helps maintain a healthy balance of stress hormones like cortisol.

5. Immune Function: Overtraining can suppress the immune system, while adequate rest supports immune health.

6. Injury Prevention: Rest allows tissues to repair, reducing the risk of overuse injuries.

Types of Rest and Recovery:

1. Passive Recovery: Complete rest, including good quality sleep and relaxation.

2. Active Recovery: Light, low-intensity exercise that promotes blood flow without adding stress to the body.

3. Sleep: Perhaps the most crucial form of recovery. Aim for 7-9 hours of quality sleep per night.

4. Nutrition: Proper nutrition, including adequate protein and carbohydrates, supports recovery processes.

5.   Hydration: Staying well-hydrated is crucial for overall health and recovery.

6.   Stress Management: Practices like meditation or deep breathing can support mental and physical recovery.

Implementing Effective Rest and Recovery:

1.   Schedule Rest Days: Include 1-2 rest days per week in your exercise plan.

2.   Practice Active Recovery: On rest days, engage in light activities like walking, yoga, or gentle swimming.

3.   Prioritize Sleep: Create a consistent sleep schedule and a relaxing bedtime routine.

4.   Use Recovery Techniques: Explore methods like foam rolling, massage, or gentle stretching.

5.   Listen to Your Body: Learn to recognize signs that you need more rest, such as persistent fatigue or decreased performance.

6.   Periodize Your Training: Plan phases of higher and lower intensity in your long-term workout schedule.

7.   Fuel Properly: Ensure you're eating enough to support your activity level and recovery needs.

8.   Stay Hydrated: Drink water consistently throughout the day, not just during workouts.

9.   Manage Stress: Incorporate stress-reduction techniques into your daily routine.

10. Consider Professional Help: Work with a trainer or coach to create a balanced program that includes adequate recovery.

Remember, rest is not laziness - it's an essential part of any successful fitness program. Balancing work and rest is key to achieving your long-term health and fitness goals.

5. Balancing Fitness Goals with Other Life Priorities

While health and fitness are important, they need to coexist with other aspects of life such as career, relationships, hobbies, and personal growth. Achieving this balance is key to long-term success and overall life satisfaction.

Strategies for Balancing Fitness with Other Priorities:

1. Define Your Priorities: Clearly identify what's most important in your life. This helps in allocating time and energy effectively.

2. Set Realistic Goals: Ensure your fitness goals are compatible with your other life commitments.

3. Integrate Fitness into Daily Life: Look for ways to incorporate movement into your regular routine, like taking stairs or walking meetings.

4. Use Time Management Techniques: Tools like calendar blocking can help you allocate time for fitness alongside other priorities.

5.   Be Flexible: Have multiple workout options of varying durations to fit different schedule scenarios.

6.   Involve Family and Friends: Make fitness a social activity to combine it with relationship time.

7.   Learn to Say No: It's okay to decline commitments that don't align with your priorities.

8.   Optimize Your Workouts: Focus on efficiency. High-Intensity Interval Training (HIIT) can provide benefits in shorter time frames.

9.   Prepare in Advance: Meal prep and laying out workout clothes can save time and reduce stress.

10.   Use Technology Wisely: Fitness apps and online workouts can provide flexibility in how and when you exercise.

11.   Practice Mindfulness: Stay present in each activity, whether it's work, family time, or exercise.

12.   Reassess Regularly: Periodically review your goals and adjust as your life circumstances change.

Handling Common Challenges:

1.   Work-Life-Fitness Balance:

- Schedule workouts like any other important appointment.

- Use lunch breaks for quick workouts or healthy meal prep.

o   Negotiate flexible work hours if possible to accommodate fitness needs.

2.   Family Responsibilities:

o   Involve family in active outings or play.

o   Use children's activities as opportunities for your own exercise (e.g., walking laps during their sports practice).

o   Communicate the importance of your health to your family and ask for their support.

3.   Social Life:

o   Suggest active social activities like hiking or dance classes.

o   Plan meals at restaurants with healthy options.

o   Learn to enjoy social events without overindulging.

4.   Personal Time:

o   Combine fitness with other personal interests (e.g., listening to audiobooks while running).

o   View exercise as self-care and personal time, not just a chore.

5.   Travel and Disrupted Routines:

- o   Have a travel workout plan that requires minimal or no equipment.

- o   Use new environments as opportunities for active exploration.

Remember, balance doesn't mean giving equal time to everything every day. It's about ensuring that over time, you're attending to all important aspects of your life, including your health and fitness. The goal is to create a sustainable lifestyle where fitness enhances, rather than detracts from, other life priorities.

6. Celebrating Non-Scale Victories

While weight loss is a common fitness goal, focusing solely on the number on the scale can be demotivating and overlook many important health improvements. Celebrating non-scale victories (NSVs) can provide motivation, reinforce positive habits, and offer a more holistic view of health and fitness progress.

Examples of Non-Scale Victories:

1.   Improved Energy Levels: Noticing you have more energy throughout the day.

2.   Better Sleep: Falling asleep more easily or waking up feeling more refreshed.

3.   Increased Strength: Being able to lift heavier weights or do more repetitions.

4.   Enhanced Endurance: Running farther or exercising for longer without fatigue.

5. Improved Flexibility: Touching your toes or achieving a deeper stretch.

6. Clothing Fit: Clothes fitting more comfortably, even if weight hasn't changed significantly.

7. Better Mood: Noticing improvements in overall mood or reduced symptoms of anxiety or depression.

8. Healthier Habits: Consistently choosing nutritious foods or maintaining a regular exercise routine.

9. Improved Health Markers: Better blood pressure, cholesterol levels, or blood sugar control.

10. Increased Confidence: Feeling more self-assured in various life situations.

11. Stress Management: Handling stress more effectively.

12. Reduced Pain: Experiencing less joint pain or back discomfort.

13. Improved Posture: Standing taller or sitting with better alignment.

14. Better Focus: Noticing improved concentration at work or in daily tasks.

15. Positive Self-Talk: Catch yourself having more positive thoughts about your body and abilities.

How to Celebrate Non-Scale Victories:

1. Keep a Victory Journal: Regularly write down NSVs you notice, no matter how small.

2.   Share Your Victories: Tell friends, family, or a support group about your NSVs to reinforce their importance.

3.   Visual Reminders: Create a vision board or progress photos to visualize non-scale improvements.

4.   Reward Yourself: Set up a reward system for achieving specific NSVs.

5.   Reflect Regularly: Take time each week to think about the positive changes you've experienced.

6.   Set Non-Scale Goals: Include NSV-related goals in your fitness plan, not just weight-related ones.

7.   Track Metrics Beyond Weight: Regularly measure things like strength, endurance, or flexibility.

8.   Celebrate Others' NSVs: Recognizing others' victories can help you appreciate your own.

The Importance of Celebrating NSVs:

Motivation: NSVs provide regular doses of motivation, even when the scale isn't moving.

Holistic Health View: They encourage a more complete picture of health beyond just weight.

Sustainable Mindset: Focusing on NSVs promotes a long-term, lifestyle change mentality.

Positive Reinforcement: Celebrating NSVs reinforces the behaviors that led to these improvements.

Mental Health: Recognizing diverse achievements can boost self-esteem and body image.

Resilience: NSVs can provide encouragement during plateaus or setbacks in weight loss.

Remember, health and fitness are about much more than a number on the scale. By recognizing and celebrating non-scale victories, you create a more positive, sustainable approach to your fitness journey. These victories reflect real improvements in your quality of life and overall health, which are ultimately more important than any number on a scale.

Long-term success in fitness and health is about more than just reaching a specific goal – it's about creating a sustainable lifestyle that supports your overall well-being. By transitioning from a dieting mentality to a lifestyle change approach, you set yourself up for lasting success. This involves not just changing what you eat or how you exercise, but shifting your entire mindset about health and fitness.

Maintaining motivation over the long haul is crucial, and this chapter has provided numerous strategies to help you stay committed to your health journey. Remember that motivation will naturally ebb and flow, and having a toolkit of motivational strategies can help you push through the challenging times.

Life is dynamic, and your fitness routine needs to be adaptable to keep up with life's changes. Whether it's a new job, a growing family, or changing health needs, having the flexibility to adjust your routine ensures that fitness remains a consistent part of your life, regardless of what changes come your way.

The importance of rest and recovery cannot be overstated. In our often fast-paced, achievement-oriented society, it's easy to overlook the value of downtime. However, proper rest is essential for physical recovery, mental refreshment, and long-term consistency in your fitness journey.

Balancing fitness goals with other life priorities is a constant juggling act, but it's essential for creating a fulfilled, well-rounded life. By integrating fitness into your daily routine and aligning it with your other priorities, you can create a sustainable, enjoyable approach to health.

Finally, celebrating non-scale victories allows you to recognize the myriad ways that your health and fitness journey is improving your life. These victories reinforce the positive changes you're making and provide motivation beyond just a number on the scale.

Remember, the goal of your fitness journey is not perfection, but progress. It's about creating a lifestyle that enhances your overall quality of life, allows you to engage fully in activities you enjoy, and supports your long-term health and well-being. By implementing the strategies discussed in this chapter, you're well on your way to not just achieving your fitness goals, but maintaining them for life.

Your journey to health and fitness is unique to you. Embrace the process, be patient with yourself, and celebrate every step forward. With consistency, adaptability, and a positive mindset, you can create a healthy lifestyle that not only helps you reach your goals but becomes an enjoyable, integral part of who you are.

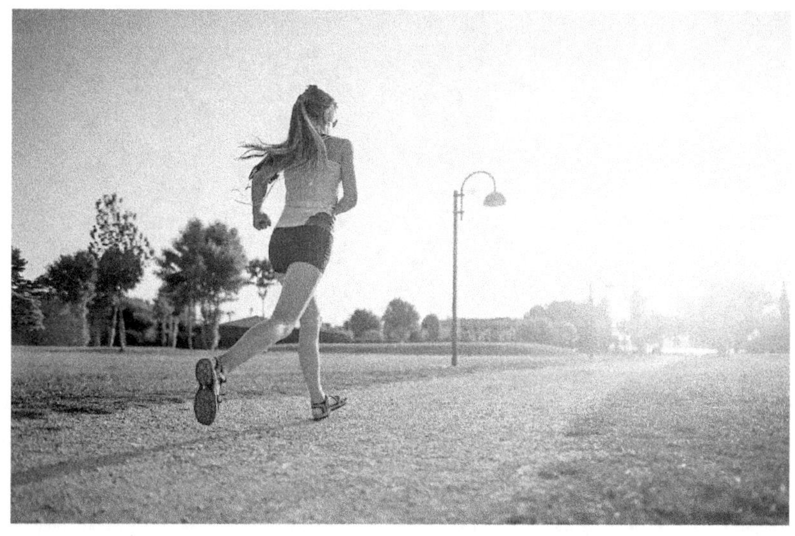

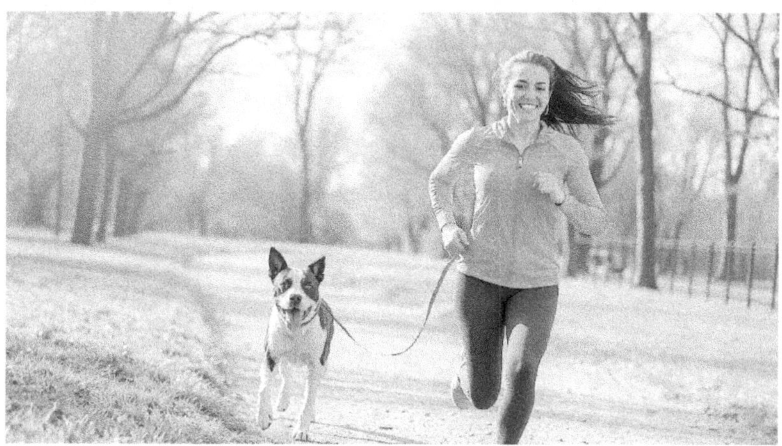

Conclusion

Your Journey to Lifelong Fitness

As we reach the end of this comprehensive guide to fitness and wellness, let's take a moment to reflect on the key points we've covered and look ahead to the exciting journey that awaits you.

Recap of Key Points

Understanding Fitness Fundamentals

We began by exploring the core components of fitness: cardiovascular endurance, muscular strength, flexibility, and body composition. Remember that a well-rounded fitness program should address all these aspects to promote overall health and well-being.

The Role of Nutrition in Fitness

Proper nutrition is the foundation of any successful fitness journey. We discussed the importance of macronutrients (proteins, carbohydrates, and fats) and micronutrients (vitamins and minerals) in fueling your body and supporting your fitness goals.

Remember, there's no one-size-fits-all diet; the key is finding a balanced, sustainable eating plan that works for you.

Exercise Types and Their Benefits

We explored various forms of exercise, including cardiovascular training, strength training, flexibility work, and high-intensity interval training (HIIT). Each type of exercise offers unique benefits, and incorporating a mix into your routine can help you achieve a well-rounded fitness level.

Creating an Effective Workout Plan

We learned about the principles of exercise programming, including progressive overload, specificity, and periodization. Remember that a good workout plan should be tailored to your individual goals, fitness level, and preferences while also being flexible enough to adapt to your changing needs.

The Importance of Rest and Recovery

We highlighted the crucial role that rest and recovery play in any fitness program. Adequate sleep, proper nutrition, and scheduled rest days are not signs of weakness but essential components of progress and injury prevention.

Overcoming Mental Barriers

We addressed common psychological obstacles to fitness, such as lack of motivation, fear of failure, and negative self-talk. Remember that your mindset is just as important as your physical effort in achieving your fitness goals.

The Role of Technology in Fitness

We explored how various technologies, from fitness apps to wearable devices, can support your fitness journey. While these tools can be helpful, remember that they should enhance, not replace, your intrinsic motivation and body awareness.

Debunking Fitness Myths

We tackled numerous myths and misconceptions in the fitness world, emphasizing the importance of evidence-based approaches over fad diets and quick fixes. Always be critical of extreme claims and seek information from reputable sources.

Adapting Fitness to Different Life Stages

We discussed how to adjust your fitness approach for different life stages and circumstances, from youth to senior years, and through various life changes. Remember that fitness is a lifelong journey that should evolve with you.

Long-term Success and Lifestyle Integration

Finally, we explored strategies for making fitness a sustainable part of your lifestyle, including how to stay motivated, adapt to life changes, and celebrate non-scale victories.

Encouragement for the Fitness Journey Ahead

As you embark on or continue your fitness journey, remember these key points:

1. Your Journey is Unique: There's no one-size-fits-all approach to fitness. What works for someone else may not work for you, and that's okay. Embrace the process of

discovering what resonates with your body, preferences, and lifestyle.

2. Progress, Not Perfection: Fitness is not about achieving a perfect body or performance. It's about consistently making choices that improve your health and well-being. Celebrate every step forward, no matter how small.

3. Embrace the Process: The joy of fitness isn't just in reaching goals but in the daily act of taking care of your body. Learn to love the process – the challenge of a tough workout, the satisfaction of making nutritious food choices, the feeling of getting stronger and more capable.

4. Be Patient and Persistent: Real, lasting changes take time. There will be ups and downs, plateaus and breakthroughs. Stay consistent, and trust that your efforts will pay off in the long run.

5. Listen to Your Body: While it's important to push yourself, it's equally crucial to respect your body's signals. Learn to distinguish between the discomfort of growth and the pain of potential injury.

6. Stay Curious and Keep Learning: The world of health and fitness is always evolving. Stay open to new information, be willing to experiment with different approaches, and never stop learning about your body and what it needs to thrive.

7. Find Your Community: Surround yourself with people who support your fitness goals. Whether it's a workout buddy, a

social media group, or a local fitness class, community can provide motivation, accountability, and fun.

8. Balance is Key: Remember that fitness is just one aspect of a fulfilling life. Strive for balance, ensuring that your fitness pursuits enhance rather than detract from other important areas of your life.

9. Be Kind to Yourself: There will be days when you don't meet your own expectations. Treat yourself with the same kindness and understanding you'd offer a good friend. Self-compassion is crucial for long-term success.

10. Celebrate Non-Scale Victories: Don't let the number on the scale be your only measure of success. Celebrate improved energy, better sleep, increased strength, enhanced mood, and all the ways fitness enriches your life.

Remember, embarking on a fitness journey is one of the most empowering decisions you can make for yourself. It's not just about changing your body; it's about enhancing your overall quality of life. Every workout, every nutritious meal, every mindful choice is an investment in your future self.

There may be challenges ahead, but you have the knowledge and tools to overcome them. Trust in your ability to adapt, grow, and persevere. Your body is capable of amazing things, and with consistent effort and a positive mindset, you can achieve more than you ever thought possible.

So, lace up those sneakers, fill up that water bottle, and step forward with confidence. Your journey to lifelong fitness starts now, and it's going to be an incredible adventure. Embrace the challenge, enjoy the process, and look forward to becoming the healthiest, strongest version of yourself.

Here's to your health, your strength, and your unwavering commitment to living your best life. The path ahead is yours to shape – make it amazing!

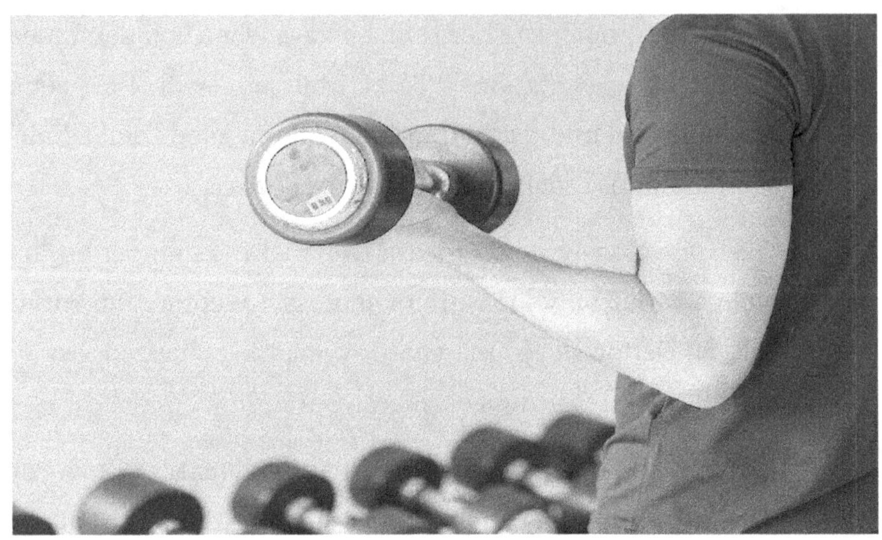

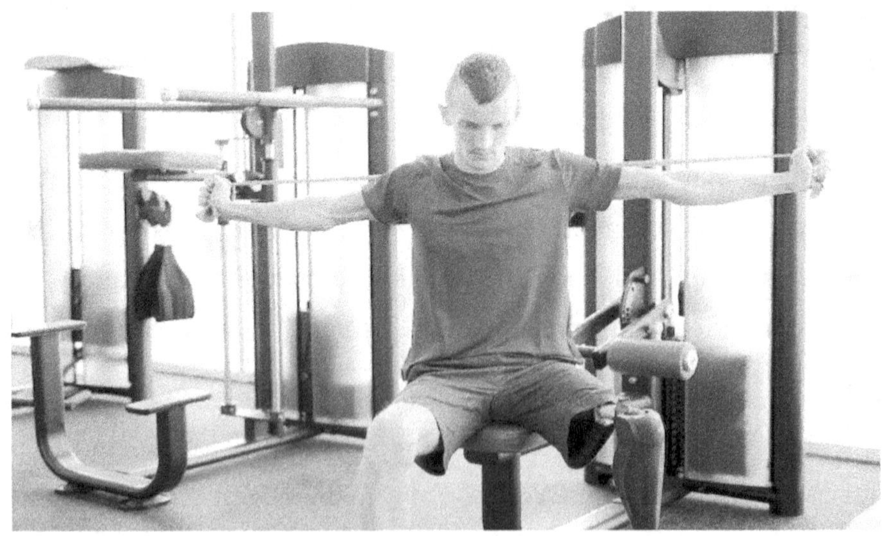

Appendices

Sample Workout Routines for Beginners

Starting a new fitness routine can be daunting, but with these beginner-friendly workouts, you'll be on your way to a healthier, stronger you in no time. Remember to warm up before each workout and cool down afterward.

1. Full Body Strength Training Routine

Perform this routine 2-3 times per week, with at least one day of rest between sessions.

1. Bodyweight Squats: 3 sets of 10-12 reps

2. Push-ups (or knee push-ups): 3 sets of 8-10 reps

3. Lunges: 3 sets of 10 reps per leg

4. Plank: 3 sets, hold for 20-30 seconds

5. Dumbbell Rows: 3 sets of 10-12 reps per arm

6. Glute Bridges: 3 sets of 12-15 reps

2. Cardio Routine for Beginners

Perform this routine 3-4 times per week.

1.   5-minute warm-up: Light walking or marching in place

2.   20 minutes of brisk walking, light jogging, or cycling at a moderate pace

3.   5-minute cool-down: Slow walk and light stretching

As you build endurance, gradually increase the duration of the main exercise portion.

3. Flexibility and Mobility Routine

Perform this routine daily or at least 3 times per week. Hold each stretch for 15-30 seconds, breathing deeply.

1.   Neck rolls

2.   Shoulder rolls

3.   Arm circles

4.   Torso twists

5.   Standing quad stretch

6.   Standing calf stretch

7.   Seated forward bend

8.   Seated spinal twist

9.   Cat-Cow stretch

10.   Child's pose

4. Beginner's HIIT Workout

Perform this routine 2-3 times per week, with rest days in between.

Perform each exercise for 30 seconds, followed by 30 seconds of rest. Repeat the circuit 3-4 times.

1.   Jumping jacks

2.   High knees

3.   Mountain climbers

4.   Bodyweight squats

5.   Burpees (without push-up)

5. Beginner's Yoga Flow

Practice this flow 2-3 times per week. Hold each pose for 3-5 breaths.

1.   Mountain pose

2.   Forward fold

3.   Plank pose

4.   Downward facing dog

5.   Warrior I (right side)

6.   Warrior II (right side)

7.   Triangle pose (right side)

8.   Repeat 5-7 on left side

9.   Child's pose

10.   Corpse pose (final relaxation)

Remember to listen to your body and modify exercises as needed. As you gain strength and confidence, gradually increase the intensity and duration of your workouts.

6. Healthy Recipe Ideas

Fueling your body with nutritious meals is crucial for supporting your fitness goals. Here are some simple, healthy recipes to get you started.

Breakfast Options

1.   Overnight Oats

Ingredients:

- 1/2 cup rolled oats

- 1/2 cup milk (dairy or plant-based)

- 1/4 cup Greek yogurt

- 1 tbsp chia seeds

- 1/2 banana, mashed

- 1/4 tsp vanilla extract

- Toppings: berries, nuts, or a drizzle of honey

Instructions: Mix all ingredients in a jar. Refrigerate overnight. Add toppings before eating.

2.   Veggie and Egg Muffins

Ingredients:

- 6 eggs
- 1/4 cup milk
- 1 cup chopped mixed vegetables (spinach, bell peppers, onions)
- 1/4 cup shredded cheese
- Salt and pepper to taste

Instructions: Whisk eggs and milk. Add vegetables, cheese, salt, and pepper. Pour into muffin tins. Bake at 350°F (175°C) for 20-25 minutes.

Lunch Ideas

1.   Quinoa and Black Bean Bowl

Ingredients:

- 1 cup cooked quinoa
- 1/2 cup black beans
- 1/4 avocado, sliced
- 1/4 cup corn
- 1/4 cup cherry tomatoes, halved
- 1 tbsp lime juice

- 1 tsp olive oil

- Salt and pepper to taste

Instructions: Combine all ingredients in a bowl. Toss with lime juice, olive oil, salt, and pepper.

2.   Greek Salad Wrap

Ingredients:

- 1 whole wheat tortilla

- 2 tbsp hummus

- 1/4 cup chopped cucumber

- 1/4 cup chopped tomatoes

- 2 tbsp crumbled feta cheese

- 1/4 cup chopped lettuce

- 2 tbsp sliced olives

- 1 tsp olive oil

- 1 tsp lemon juice

Instructions: Spread hummus on tortilla. Layer with vegetables, feta, and olives. Drizzle with olive oil and lemon juice. Roll up and serve.

Dinner Recipes

1.   Baked Salmon with Roasted Vegetables

Ingredients:

- 4 oz salmon fillet

- 1 cup mixed vegetables (broccoli, carrots, zucchini)

  - 1 tbsp olive oil

  - 1 tsp lemon juice

  - 1 clove garlic, minced

  - Salt and pepper to taste

Instructions: Preheat oven to 400°F (200°C). Place salmon and vegetables on a baking sheet. Drizzle with olive oil, lemon juice, and sprinkle with garlic, salt, and pepper. Bake for 15-20 minutes.

2.   Turkey and Vegetable Stir-Fry

Ingredients:

  - 4 oz ground turkey

  - 2 cups mixed vegetables (bell peppers, snap peas, carrots)

  - 1 tbsp soy sauce

  - 1 tsp sesame oil

  - 1 clove garlic, minced

  - 1 tsp grated ginger

  - 1/2 cup cooked brown rice

Instructions: Cook turkey in a pan. Add vegetables, garlic, and ginger. Stir-fry until vegetables are tender-crisp. Add soy sauce and sesame oil. Serve over brown rice.

Snack Ideas

1. Apple slices with almond butter

2. Greek yogurt with berries and a drizzle of honey

3. Carrot sticks with hummus

4. Hard-boiled egg with whole grain crackers

5. Handful of mixed nuts and dried fruit

Remember to adjust portion sizes based on your individual calorie needs and fitness goals. Stay hydrated by drinking plenty of water throughout the day.

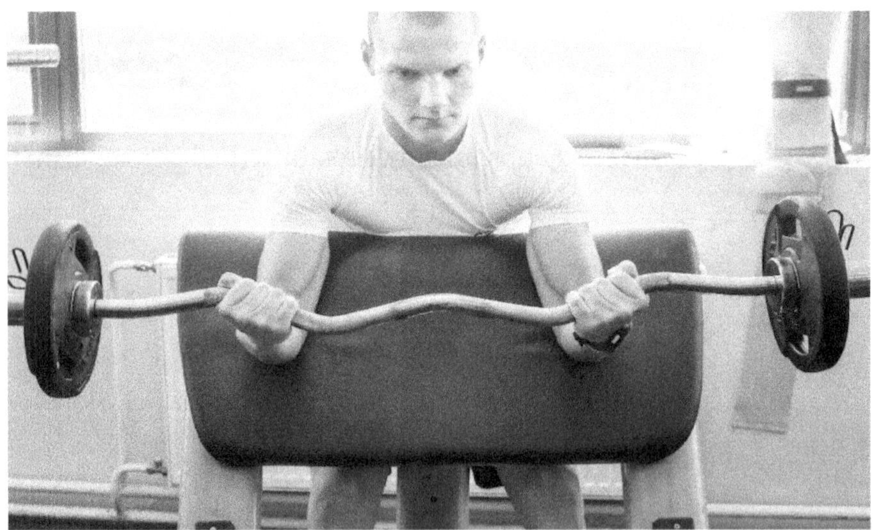

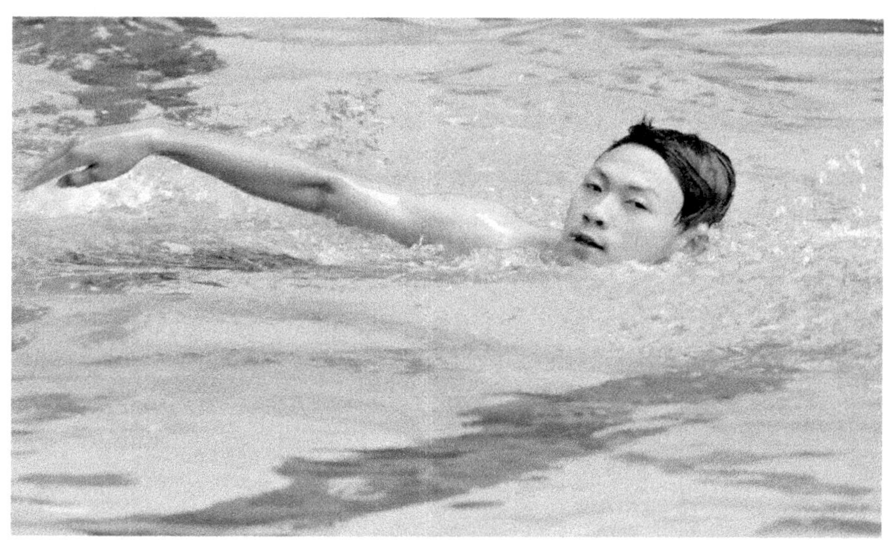

Workout Glossary

Understanding common fitness terms can help you navigate your workout routines more effectively. Here's a glossary of frequently used workout terminology:

1. **AMRAP**: As Many Rounds (or Reps) As Possible. A workout structure where you perform as many rounds of a circuit or as many repetitions of an exercise as you can within a set time frame.

2. **BMI (Body Mass Index)**: A measure that uses your height and weight to work out if your weight is healthy. While useful for general population studies, it has limitations for individuals, especially athletes.

3. **DOMS (Delayed Onset Muscle Soreness)**: The muscle pain and stiffness that occurs 24-48 hours after a workout, especially after introducing new exercises or increasing intensity.

4. **Drop Set**: A technique where you perform an exercise to failure, then immediately reduce the weight and continue for more repetitions.

5.   **EMOM (Every Minute On the Minute)**: A workout structure where you perform a specific task at the start of every minute for a set duration.

6.   **HIIT (High-Intensity Interval Training)**: A training technique that involves intense bursts of exercise followed by short recovery periods.

7.   **Isometric Exercise**: An exercise where muscles contract and hold a static position without visible movement.

8.   **LISS (Low-Intensity Steady State)**: Cardio performed at a low intensity for an extended duration, like a long, slow jog.

9.   **Macros (Macronutrients)**: The three main nutrients your body needs in large quantities: proteins, carbohydrates, and fats.

10.   **One-Rep Max (1RM)**: The maximum weight you can lift for a single repetition of an exercise with proper form.

11.   **Plyometrics**: Exercises that involve rapid stretching and contracting of muscles to increase power, often involving jumping movements.

12.   **Progressive Overload**: Gradually increasing the weight, frequency, or number of repetitions in your strength training routine to continuously challenge your muscles.

13.   **Rep (Repetition)**: One complete motion of an exercise.

14.   **Set**: A group of repetitions performed without resting.

15. **Spotting**: Assisting another person during a weight training exercise to help them lift heavier weights and prevent injury.

16. **Superset**: Performing two exercises back-to-back with little to no rest in between.

17. **TABATA**: A form of HIIT that involves 20 seconds of all-out effort followed by 10 seconds of rest, repeated for 4 minutes.

18. **Target Heart Rate**: A heart rate range that ensures your heart is being exercised and conditioned but not overworked.

19. **VO2 Max**: The maximum rate of oxygen consumption measured during incremental exercise. It's an indicator of cardiovascular fitness and aerobic endurance.

20. **WOD (Workout of the Day)**: A term popularized by CrossFit, referring to the workout prescribed for that day.

21. **Compound Exercise**: An exercise that works multiple muscle groups simultaneously, such as squats or push-ups.

22. **Isolation Exercise**: An exercise that targets a single muscle group, such as bicep curls.

23. **Eccentric**: The lengthening phase of a muscle contraction, like lowering the weight during a bicep curl.

24. **Concentric**: The shortening phase of a muscle contraction, like lifting the weight during a bicep curl.

25. **RPE (Rate of Perceived Exertion)**: A scale used to measure the intensity of your exercise based on how hard you feel your body is working.

26. **Tempo**: The speed at which you perform an exercise, often broken down into the time taken for the eccentric, isometric, and concentric phases.

27. **Functional Training**: Exercises that mimic everyday movements to improve overall functionality in daily life.

28. **Periodization**: A systematic planning of athletic or physical training, typically involving progressive cycling of various aspects of a training program during a specific period.

29. **ROM (Range of Motion)**: The full movement potential of a joint, usually its range of flexion and extension.

30. **Fartlek**: A training technique, particularly for runners, that involves varying the intensity of exercise within a single session.

31. **Burpee**: A full-body exercise that involves a squat thrust and a jump.

32. **Circuit Training**: A form of workout where you cycle through several exercises targeting different muscle groups with minimal rest in between.

33. **Cool Down**: A period of light exercise following more intense activity to allow the body to gradually transition to a resting or near-resting state.

34. **Core**: The muscles of your midsection, including the abdominals, obliques, and lower back muscles.

35. **Cross-Training**: Incorporating various types of exercise in your routine to improve overall fitness and reduce the risk of injury.

36. **Foam Rolling**: A self-myofascial release technique using a foam roller to massage muscles and improve flexibility.

37. **Form**: The proper posture and movement pattern for a particular exercise.

38. **Gains**: Improvements in muscle size, strength, or overall fitness.

39. **Interval Training**: Alternating periods of high-intensity exercise with periods of lower-intensity exercise or rest.

40. **Kettlebell**: A cast-iron weight shaped like a ball with a handle, used for various exercise movements.

41. **Lactic Acid**: A substance produced in muscles during intense exercise that can contribute to the burning sensation felt during workouts.

42. **Mobility**: The ability to move a joint through its full range of motion with control.

43. **Plateau**: A period where you stop seeing progress in your fitness goals despite consistent effort.

44. **Power**: The ability to exert maximum force in the shortest time possible.

45. **Resistance Training**: Any form of exercise that causes the muscles to contract against an external resistance.

46. **Reps in Reserve (RIR)**: The number of additional repetitions you could perform in a set before reaching failure.

47. **Stability**: The ability to maintain control of joint movement or position.

48. **Stretching**: Deliberately lengthening muscles to increase flexibility and range of motion.

49. **Warm-Up**: A period of light exercise before a workout to gradually rev up your cardiovascular system and increase blood flow to your muscles.

50. **Yoga**: A practice that combines physical postures, breathing techniques, and meditation.

Understanding these terms will help you better navigate workout instructions, fitness articles, and conversations with trainers or workout partners. Remember, if you encounter a term you're not familiar with, don't hesitate to ask for clarification. Continuous learning is part of the fitness journey!

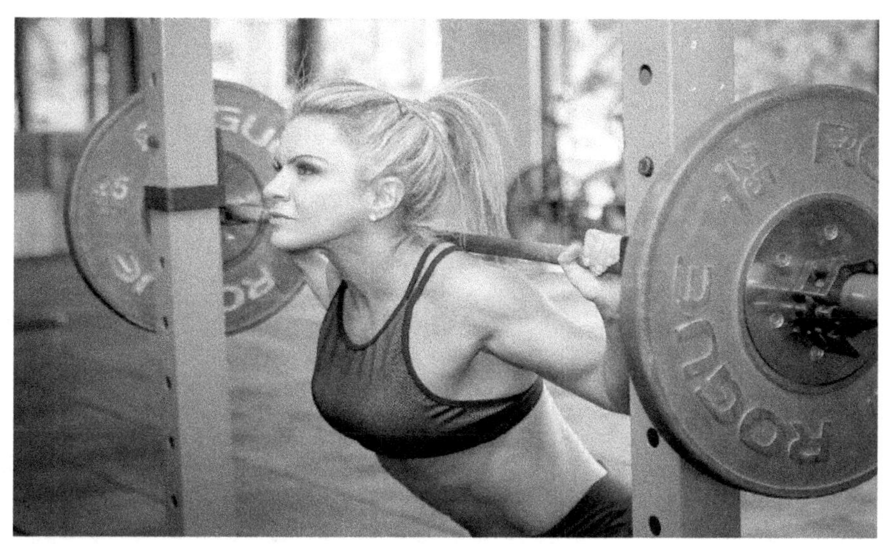

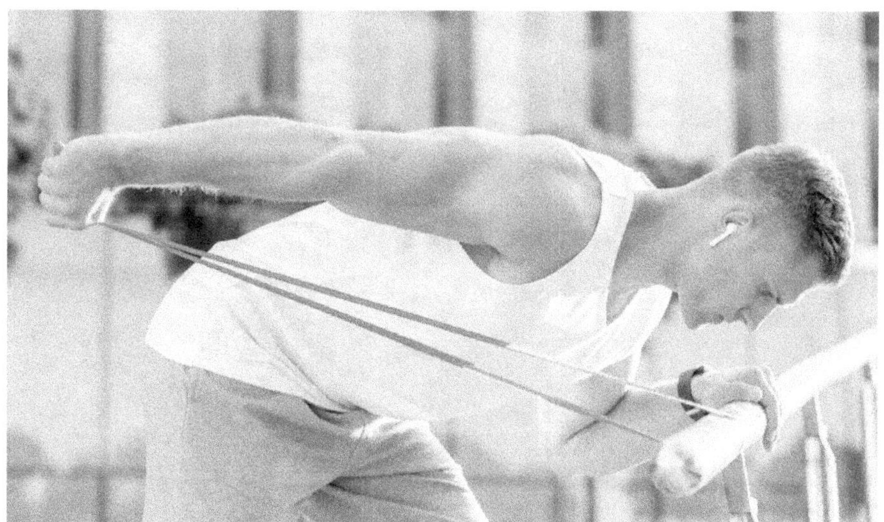